Positive
Mind,
Healthy
Heart

Also by Joseph C. Piscatella

Don't Eat Your Heart Out Cookbook

Choices for a Healthy Heart

Controlling Your Fat Tooth

The Fat-Gram Counter

The Fat-Gram Guide to Restaurant Food

Fat-Proof Your Child

Take a Load Off Your Heart

The Healthy Heart Cookbook

The Road to a Healthy Heart Runs Through the Kitchen

Positive Mind, Healthy Heart

Take Charge of Your Cardiac Health, One Day at a Time

JOSEPH C. PISCATELLA

WORKMAN PUBLISHING • NEW YORK

As always, to my wife Bernie, with love and gratitude.
Sharing a lifetime with you has been my main motivation.

Copyright © 2010 by Joseph C. Piscatella
All rights reserved. No portion of this book may be reproduced—
mechanically, electronically, or by any other means, including
photocopying—without written permission of the publisher. Published
simultaneously in Canada by Thomas Allen & Son Limited.

Library of Congress Cataloging-in-Publication Data is available.
ISBN 978-0-7611-5457-0

We are grateful for permission to reprint material from the
following sources: *The Word for Today* by Bob Gass (United Christian
Broadcasters); *Rebuilding the Front Porch of America* by Patrick Overton
(Columbia College, Columbia, MO, 1997); and *Footprints: Images and
Reflections of God's Presence in Our Lives* by Margaret Fishback Powers
(HarperCollins Canada, Scarborough, Ontario, Canada, 2002).

Workman books are available at special discounts when purchased in
bulk for premiums and sales promotions as well as for fund-raising or
educational use. Special editions or book excerpts also can be created
to specification. For details, contact the Special Sales Director at the
address below.

Workman Publishing Company, Inc.
225 Varick Street
New York, NY 10014-4381
www.workman.com

Printed in the United States of America
First printing January 2010
10 9 8 7 6 5 4 3 2 1

Contents

Foreword
by Bernie Piscatella

My husband, Joe, has written 10 books about cardiac health and lifestyle habits. I contributed all the recipes (more than a thousand of them!) and lots of constructive criticism, but Joe is definitely the author. So why am I, the author's wife, writing the foreword to his most recent book? Simply put: Joe feels awkward telling you the details of the story himself. And he certainly doesn't want to brag about the mental attitude that has allowed him to stick with a heart-healthy plan for more than three decades. I'm going to do it for him.

Here's the story: In 1977, at age 32, we went through coronary bypass surgery. Joe had the actual surgery, but I felt as if I were right there with him on the operating table, sharing each step of that terrifying procedure. Through his recovery and the decades since, it has always felt like *our* surgery.

We lived in Tacoma, Washington, and had two wonderful children—Anne, age six, and Joe, age four. A consciously healthy lifestyle had taken a backseat to other priorities like school, carpool, volunteering and supporting Joe's work. Besides, we had always been in good health. Serious diseases such as heart disease and cancer happened to other people. Sure, we knew that Joe's cholesterol was too high, that we both could stand to lose a few pounds, that our exercise regimen was sporadic and that, like most Americans, we lived with a chronic stress caused by never having enough time. We talked about living healthier, but doing something about it—that was for tomorrow. Then I found out that you can't have a tomorrow if you don't have a today.

For about a month, Joe had been complaining about shortness of breath and a pain in his chest that came on when he warmed up to play tennis. He described the pain as "dull, more like a feeling of fullness or pressure," and it would usually disappear by the end of the warm-up. He ignored it, hoping it would just go away. Then one day it stayed with him through two hours of play. I made him call our family doctor, who said he should come in right away. Neither of us was worried, because Joe had had an annual physical four months earlier and the results were excellent.

Joe's exam indicated that his lungs were just fine. "But as long as you're here," the doctor said, "let's do an electrocardiogram." The EKG indicated a very serious heart problem: an obstruction of a coronary artery. "I want you to see a cardiologist right now, today," said the doctor. "In fact, I'll drive you. I don't want you behind the wheel of a car." Now, *that* got Joe's attention. He spent the next hour undergoing a thorough cardiac workup that included an exercise stress test. The results were not good; the cardiologist recommended an immediate coronary angiography, an X-ray of the coronary arteries.

At that point, Joe called home. He danced around the topic, trying not to alarm me, but he finally had to get to the point. "They want to look at my coronary arteries," he said. "I don't think it's any big deal, but you might want to drop the kids off at your mom's and come on down to the hospital."

I got there just as Joe was being wheeled into the catheterization lab. We met up again in the recovery room. "Joe has coronary heart disease, a buildup of blockages in three coronary arteries," the cardiologist told us. "It looks pretty aggressive. He has two blockages better than 50%, and one that has closed about 95% of the artery. This is life-threatening. I recommend bypass surgery within the next few days. He's a heart attack waiting to happen."

Joe tried to be calm and logical (for my benefit, I'm sure) as we discussed the options, but I was gripped by pure, stomach-churning fear. Old age was something I'd looked forward to sharing with Joe. What would happen to the kids and me if he wasn't around? I had to face the fact that his death not only *could* happen in the near future, but probably *would* happen as a result of the time bomb inside his chest. Over the next hour, the doctor explained how coronary heart disease progresses, what would happen in the surgery, how the heart-lung machine works and the risks involved. With all that information in our heads, we made the hard decision: Joe would undergo bypass surgery in two days.

On the drive home, we tried to shore up each other by focusing on mundane issues. "You call the insurance agent. I'll check with our attorney about the will and power of attorney." "Who will call our parents?" "What do we tell the children?" But when we got home, and all through the night, we clung to each other.

The next day was a kind of sleepwalk as we took care of life's details, reassured the kids and placed them with relatives. One thing sticks out in my memory, though. Joe and I had a running joke about how expensive dentistry had become. I got my teeth cleaned four times a year, but two times was the max for Joe. "I'm too frugal," he'd say. Well, he kept a dental appointment that he'd made for that day, and when he returned I voiced my fear: "Do you think you won't make it through the surgery?" His answer was pure Joe: "Do you think I'd waste money getting my teeth cleaned if I thought I was going to die tomorrow?" Nothing could have given me more confidence.

We headed to the hospital in the afternoon, since the surgery was scheduled for six o'clock the next morning. Joe settled into his room and had all his tests done. Then, after an orderly shaved his chest, we had nothing to do but wait. Luckily, it was the night of the major league All-Star baseball game, so we put the TV on. Before we knew it, people started to arrive. Friends, family, neighbors . . . soon the room was overflowing with laughter and friendship as everyone watched the game.

In the fourth inning, Joe received a telephone call from Ron Cey, the Los Angeles Dodgers third baseman. He was playing that night, but he had heard about our situation from his father, who had a service station in our neighborhood, and wanted to wish Joe good luck. After they talked, other National League players got on the phone and also wished him well. For a true baseball fan, as Joe was and is, nothing could have been better. That was the night I became a National League fan!

Finally, the cardiac surgeon arrived and shooed everyone away. "Be sure to get a good night's rest," he said.

"Don't worry about me," Joe replied. "*You* be sure to get a good night's rest!"

The surgery seemed to take forever. I sat in the waiting room with my sister and brother-in-law, trying to keep my thoughts positive while fearing the worst. Finally, after five hours, the surgeon came out and told us that all had gone well and Joe was in recovery. We found him in intensive care, still not conscious, with multiple tubes running out of his body. I was so happy to see him alive, yet so sad that he had to go through all this. He just didn't look like my Joe.

At a certain point, the doctors and nurses were happy with his progress and told us to get some dinner and go home to rest. We headed out to a waterfront restaurant, ordered a bottle of wine and drank to Joe's health. We didn't know that a leak had sprung at the bypass site and blood was filling the pericardium, the heart's protective sack. The pressure was putting Joe's life at risk. The hospital called the restaurant to tell us that Joe was on his way back into surgery; I got there just in time to see him. "He won't die, will he?" I asked the surgeon. "There's a chance that he will," he said. "We'll do the best we can."

. . . .

A week after surgery, Joe was home. He was happy to
be alive and with his family again, but he was filled with
concern about the future. Bypass had not "cured" him. As
the surgeon had counseled, "You had heart disease the day
before surgery, you had heart disease the day after surgery
and you have heart disease today. The surgery took away
the pain and the threat of an imminent heart attack, but it
did not remove the disease."

This sobering fact was instrumental in our desire to
find a course of action that would allow us to manage the
disease, to arrest its progression. There were no statin
drugs back then. No beta-blockers or stents. And very little
information about managing heart disease. But Joe knew
that his cholesterol was a key issue, so he searched out a
nationally known specialist for advice. We got more than we
bargained for. "My cholesterol is over 250," Joe told him.
"Should I change my diet? Do more exercise?"

"Don't bother," the specialist replied. "You have an
aggressive form of coronary heart disease at an early
age. Frankly, I'd be surprised if you live to be 40. The
chances of you seeing your children graduate from high
school are slim."

His bedside manner certainly left a lot to be desired,
but we took him seriously. At first, I watched Joe mope
around aimlessly, but then common sense told me that
doing *something* had to be better for his (and my) mental
health than doing *nothing*. So I got up my courage and tried
to put it all into perspective for him: "It's true, you can't

change the cards you were dealt. But you can change the way you play those cards. And we're going to do everything possible to eat healthier and exercise more effectively to even up the odds. It's the only chance we have."

And so we committed ourselves to a healthier way of living. The problem was, there was no road map for what to do or how to do it. In an effort to eat better, I cleared out the "unhealthy food" from our kitchen cabinets. But I had no idea what constituted "healthy food." Joe's first week home, I made the same lunch—a turkey sandwich on cardboard-like bread—for three days running. On the third day, Joe spoke up: "Bernie, I may have survived the surgery, but I don't think I'll survive another lunch!"

A couple of months later, Joe bought a pair of running shoes (the original blue-and-yellow Nike waffles) and devised his own exercise program (there was no cardiac rehabilitation program in our area). As he was out walking, he got a sharp pain in his side and thought it was the start of a heart attack. "I thought they would find me by the mailbox," he said, "clutching my American Express bill." It turned out to be a stitch.

Two steps forward and one step back. That was our dance for the next year as we tried to institute and maintain a heart-healthy lifestyle. But by year's end Joe's exercise had become a daily routine and I felt more comfortable in the kitchen, preparing healthier recipes—many of which tasted better than the original versions. And Joe's cardiac markers—his cholesterol, weight and blood pressure—were better than ever.

Impressed with our progress, Joe's doctor asked him to write down what we were doing and how we were doing it so he could share the information with other patients. The result was the *Don't Eat Your Heart Out Cookbook,* one of the first books in the country to deal with diet, exercise and cholesterol. It was endorsed by many heart experts—the legendary Dr. Denton Cooley among them—and became a national bestseller. Over the next three decades, we would collaborate on many more books on healthy living and Joe would become a recognized expert on cardiac health and lifestyle.

More important, our healthy way of living worked. In 2009, to celebrate the 32nd anniversary of his bypass surgery, Joe hiked Mount Rainier with me. He is now one of the oldest living bypass survivors in the country, perhaps the world. His current cardiac markers show that he is in better health now than he was in 1977. His heart disease has actually reversed itself.

As a result, we've experienced the joy of seeing our daughter and son graduate from high school, college, law school and graduate school; of Joe walking our daughter down the aisle and making a toast at our son's wedding; of celebrating 42 years of marriage; of gathering with family at Joe's 65th birthday and presenting him with a bottle of his favorite wine from 1977, the year of his surgery; and of buying our four grandchildren their first baseball gloves.

And that brings us to the real point of Joe's story: how he has successfully kept with the program for more than 30 years. No matter what the situation, through the ups and downs of life, he has stayed committed to healthy living. Let me give you an example. In order to perform bypass surgery, the surgeon has to split the breastbone to get to the heart. This often produces some distress for several months after the surgery, and that's how it was for Joe (his chest, he said, could predict rain). By the sixth or seventh month his chest felt fine, but then he was in a car accident. His small sports car was violently rear-ended and pushed into the back of a stationary truck, and his breastbone was broken along the lines of the surgery. Needless to say, it was extremely painful, but that didn't keep Joe from his daily run. The day after he returned from the hospital, I found him taping up his chest with an elastic bandage. "I need to take a slow jog," he said. I tried to talk him out of it, but he told me, "When I was in the hospital, I thought about never being able to jog again—what I wouldn't give for just one more run. Well, I'm lucky enough to have many more runs, and the first one is today."

That's Joe. In the first section of this book, he sets out six simple principles to help *you* succeed in living healthy and fit for a lifetime. The second part is a collection of 365 of his favorite motivations, inspiration stories, quotes and health tips. They are what keep Joe focused on change, and our hope is that they'll do the same for you. Remember, it is only what your mind sees—whether it's taking a brisk walk or making a healthy choice for lunch—that your body can perform.

PART ONE

The Yogi Principle

*"What you do today can
improve all your tomorrows."*

—RALPH MARSTEN

Growing up in Connecticut, I was a die-hard Yankee fan. I followed the team religiously, knew players and managers from the early days, celebrated World Series victories, hated the Red Sox and lived for those trips with my father and brother to Yankee Stadium. Like most fans back then, I was crazy for Mickey Mantle, Roger Maris, Whitey Ford and Bobby Richardson—the guys who played exceptionally well but also looked the part of Yankee "supermen" in the tradition of Lou Gehrig and Joe DiMaggio. But I always had a special place in my heart for Yogi Berra.

Yogi presented a paradox. On one hand, he was a fabulous baseball player. But on the other, he didn't resemble a big-league player at all. Of just medium height with a stocky body and, let's say, a less than classically handsome face, Yogi lacked DiMaggio's grace, Mantle's power and Maris's all-American good looks. He simply didn't carry himself like an elite athlete. But with one swing of the bat he would drive in the runs to beat you; with one throw from his powerful arm, your chance of stealing second base had just disappeared. And no catcher ever called better games. He was a winner.

He still is. His unique views on life—his "Yogi-isms"—continue to mystify as they enlighten: *"If you come to a fork in the road, take it." "It ain't over till it's over." "The future ain't what it used to be."*

My favorite Yogi-ism is his answer to a question on how to be successful at the major league level: *"Baseball is 90% mental—the other half is physical."* Like many of Yogi's quotes, this doesn't make sense until you ponder it for a bit. Then you begin to see his wisdom: A positive mental attitude is at least as important as the physical tools you bring to the game. What your mind sees, be it positive or negative, becomes your reality. What Yogi knew by instinct, many scientific studies have found to be factual.

Let me give you an example from my own experience with golf. How many times have I set up to take a shot, seen the ball in my mind's eye take flight and land in a bunker, and then done in reality what I've already done in my mind? My negative thoughts produced a negative result. But when Phil Mickelson plays the round in his head before he steps to the first tee, he visualizes each shot as perfectly placed. Guess who plays better golf?

Not everyone can be a major league ballplayer or a PGA golfer, but we all can use a positive mental attitude—what I call the Yogi Principle—to improve our performance and our lives. After my coronary bypass surgery, my first step was to do research and collect information on heart-healthy living. The prescription was clear enough: eat better, manage stress and move my body more. That was the plan. But I soon found that information alone, even when part of a plan, does not bring success. Cognitive understanding does not always lead to behavior change. If it did, we would be a nation of nonsmokers.

I started out fine. I ate more vegetables and less red meat, took a morning jog or after-dinner walk, made time to de-stress by listening to music. But then a cheeseburger would creep into my diet, or a favorite television show would preempt my walk, or I would run out of time to take time for myself. Why was this turning out to be so hard?

I learned that I wasn't the only one to have trouble. National Institutes of Health data showed that up to 50% of bypass patients abandoned their low-fat diets within six months of surgery. These patients had received information on healthy eating from doctors, dietitians and cardiac rehabilitation professions, and had experienced a never-to-be-forgotten surgery. Yet just a short six months later, with their chests barely healed, they were back to chicken nuggets and fries.

That's where I found myself. Contemplating change was the easy part. Taking action and maintaining the change over time was elusive. That's because my thinking was so negative. Instead of solutions, I visualized problems and roadblocks.

It was then that I discovered the Yogi Principle: See the positive results in your mind to be successful in your actions. This was a complete turnaround for me. No longer limited by fear of failure, I began to think of new ways to solve problems. My good friend Dr. Barry Franklin, director of the Cardiac Rehabilitation Program and Exercise Laboratories at William Beaumont Hospital in Michigan, makes this point by telling a story about two salesmen sent to the Australian outback to sell shoes. They each encounter barefoot Aborigines in their travels. The first salesman e-mails back to his company: "No potential for sales here. The people don't wear shoes. I'm coming home." The second salesman looks at things differently. His e-mail? "Wonderful potential here. The people don't wear shoes."

Now, don't get me wrong. Despite what many gurus preach, just thinking positively doesn't cut it. Everyone who accomplishes something, whether it's hitting a sales goal or becoming a top-tier surgeon, accomplishes it the same way: *by taking action.* Positive people simply have an edge because they believe, they *know,* that the object of their desire is attainable. When I started to collect the information I needed to make healthy changes, I wanted to develop a "can do" attitude. But I soon found that such an attitude was all about *potential.* It wasn't until I had established a "will do" attitude that change really began to take place.

Building on the Foundation: Six Principles for Success

Once you start your journey down the road to health by employing a positive mental attitude and a "will do" mind-set, you'll be ready to use six basic principles that will assist you in achieving your diet, exercise and stress management goals.

1. DEVELOP RESILIENCY

Everyday life is filled with events that can knock any of us down. No one is immune, but the way a person reacts to a blow can be 180 degrees apart from how somebody else responds. One person can be devastated by losing a job, while another takes a deep breath and moves on. One person simply collapses under the weight of his troubles, while his neighbor actively looks for a way to get through them and even thrive. That's the resilient guy I want to focus on—the fellow who, whatever comes his way, manages to keep control of his thoughts, feelings, focus and actions. He's the person who, when knocked down, bounces back.

By way of example, let me tell you about Jim and Tom, a couple of cardiac patients in their mid-fifties whom I met after giving a talk at a hospital. They worked for the same company and had undergone bypass surgery in the same month, but there the similarity ended. Jim was doing wonderfully. He viewed the changes in his life—healthy eating, regular exercise—as welcome arrivals. He was thankful that the surgery had given him a second chance and additional years of life, and was determined to live those years to the fullest. Excited about his future, he could visualize himself growing and prospering. When I met him, he was planning an 80-mile backpacking trip into the mountains with his sons. For Jim, lifestyle change was a beginning, a way to demonstrate his new resiliency.

Tom was as far removed from Jim's state of mind as anyone could be. Soon after the operation, he crawled into a mental fetal position. *My life is over,* he thought. In his mind, he was an old and frail person with a bad heart, and that became his reality. He grew more fearful, unwilling to try new things, socially isolated. Though still alive, he was a cardiac casualty, and he left the rehabilitation program without completing it. Researchers investigating how the mind-body connection affects health have become increasingly interested in people like Jim. Studies show that resilient people often share distinctive habits, including a positive attitude that helps them shape a "hardy" personality. In other words, you can develop a resilient response to any situation as the result of the way you think. Resilient people look at each situation as an opportunity for growth, often by focusing on immediate issues rather than far-reaching ones.

Early on in my attempt to practice healthy lifestyle habits, I came across a study that examined the responses of executives laid off in a corporate restructuring. Many were career men in midlife whose entire working lives had been with one company. The study described the stress and anxiety (and sometimes depression) that many of them exhibited. But what I found really interesting was that some people not only accepted the change, but flourished as a result of it. Each of this latter group of executives had four particularly helpful character traits:

- A sense of control. They felt that they could shape events and turn situations, even bad ones, to their advantage.

- A commitment to life. They believed that their actions were worth doing at full tilt since their lives were of use —to themselves, their families and society.

- Love of a challenge. They demonstrated a willingness to accept and anticipate change as natural and exciting, not threatening.

- A sense of purpose. This helped them overcome obstacles in their path.

Can you learn resiliency? The answer is yes, if you have a positive mental attitude.

2. DEVELOP PERSEVERANCE

Simply thinking positive thoughts will not get the job done. Whatever you call it—perseverance, stick-to-it-iveness, commitment—you need to not only take action but keep on doing it. That's the difference between "can do" and "will do," and it's the only way you can develop the new habits you desire.

Here's a favorite story of mine. A sales manager is firing up his people. "Did the Wright brothers quit?" he asks.

"No!" they answer in unison.

"Did Rocky quit?"

"No!" they yell.

"Did Lance Armstrong quit?"

"No!" they bellow.

"Did Thorndike McKester quit?"

A long confused silence. Then a salesperson shouts from the audience: "Who in the world is Thorndike McKester? Nobody's ever heard of him."

The sales manager shouts back: "Of course not. He quit!"

You need to just keep plugging on, no matter what happens in the course of any particular day. It is said that when his crew grew discouraged after three weeks at sea, Columbus urged them on by shouting, *"Adelante! Adelante!"*— "Sail on! Sail on!" Persevering means stopping not when you lose heart but when the task is done. As Robert Strauss, diplomat and adviser to U.S. presidents, once remarked, "It's a little like wrestling a gorilla. You don't quit when you're tired. You quit when the gorilla is tired."

Let me tell you, this is easier said than done, particularly when success eludes us. But failure, which is part of the human condition, does not have to equal weakness. In fact, it can motivate growth—if you stick with the program. This is where your ability to paint a positive mental picture comes in. If you're trying to eat healthy but fall off the wagon with a hot fudge sundae, your thought might be *Can't I do anything right? I'm always eating something wrong. I'm just a loser!* That message triggers emotional stress and you give up. But what if you say to yourself: *That sundae was great! Everyone deserves a now-and-then indulgence. Tomorrow I'll be back to eating healthy again.* That response strengthens your resolve and, ultimately, your ability to persevere.

3. TAKE RESPONSIBILITY FOR YOURSELF AND YOUR ACTIONS

Too often the answer to the question "Who or what is responsible for your health?" is "my doctor" or "my genes." As a game show host might say, "Wrong answer!" Sure, heredity plays a part in our health, and so do the people who take care of us. But what we do to and for our bodies is a personal responsibility.

After my surgery, I visited my cardiologist. I had done some research on diet and heart disease, and now I was ready to take action. "My diet is a critical factor in recovery, isn't it?" I asked.

"Yes, that's true," he replied. "Your cholesterol and triglyceride levels are too high and you need to lose a few pounds. Healthy eating will help."

"What are we going to do about that?" I asked.

"Darned if I know," he said. "I'm a doctor and I understand disease. If you have another blockage, come back and see me. But what you're talking about is not disease; it's health. And frankly, health is not my field."

I was stung by his comments and so angry that I could hardly speak. Fortunately, he had to leave the exam room for a call, which gave me time to cool down.

While it's true that no doctor today would say such a thing (remember, this was more than 30 years ago), I was grateful for his directness. He could do a lot for me—direct me to a cardiac rehabilitation program, give me books to read, line me up with a dietitian and lend me his support—but he couldn't change my lifestyle. He knew that. He also knew that I was looking for a pill or a prescription, a quick fix for my problem, and that I wanted to make him the person in charge. His dismissive tone literally shocked me into a profound understanding of my responsibility. It was *my* heart, *my* life, *my* diet, *my* health. The decisions and actions were mine, too.

4. SET REALISTIC GOALS

Whether you're developing a financial strategy or planning a vacation, to get what you want you must first know what you want. You must have a goal. As Yogi Berra liked to say, "If you don't know where you're going, you'll end up somewhere else." The same holds true in constructing a healthy lifestyle. Set an explicit goal ("I'm going to lose 20 pounds") rather than a general one ("I'd like to lose some weight"). This provides direction and a heightened sense of purpose, and will give you both short-term motivation and a long-term vision. As you achieve your goals, the feeling of success will keep you on track.

It's particularly important to commit goals to writing. Written goals demand clarity, conditions, a time frame and a strategy—a process that makes the goals real. The act of writing makes it easier to prioritize, to focus your time and energy on what's important, to review what you've done and measure your results.

Keep your goals realistic, achievable. Losing 20 pounds may be appropriate, but expecting to do it in a month is not. You may have to change your lifestyle in a number of ways, but don't tackle them all at once. In short, timing is everything. Starting a healthy diet, reducing stress, beginning an exercise program, giving up smoking—to try to do all this at the same time is to invite frustration and failure.

Instead, try to see change as a steady progression. Walking today *will* lead to power walking or jogging tomorrow. Research suggests that it takes about two to six months to accomplish significant changes and turn them into habits. During that time, you should not feel pressured to rush or succeed. This isn't a race; it's about how you want to live for the rest of your life.

5. GET STRAIGHT INFORMATION

We are awash in information about healthy living, but unfortunately much of it is *mis*information, designed to sell a product, a book or a DVD. In three decades of managing heart disease, I've learned to rely only on tested information from reliable sources. When the American Heart Association, the American Dietetic Association or the USDA publishes dietary guidelines, I pay close attention.

The impact of positive thinking on cardiac health is grounded in credible science. Studies published in *Circulation* and the *Archives of General Psychiatry* suggest that a positive, optimistic outlook can reduce depression, anxiety and coronary inflamation—all serious risk factors. Says Dr. Leo Pozuelo of the Cleveland Clinic, "There is a growing amount of literature showing that a positive, optimistic attitude can decrease the incidence of heart disease and extend good health and longer lives. One of the most important contributions to heart health, it seems, is a healthy brain."

6. HAVE FAITH

I have always believed that faith in a higher power provides comfort and resolve as we make our journey to good health. Now many scientific studies have reached the same conclusion. A 28-year survey conducted by Yale University found that people who worship regularly are happier, enjoy better health and live longer than those who don't. The people of faith in this study had lower blood pressure, less stress and greater immunity to disease. One of the interviewers asked an 80-year-old woman, who was exercising on a treadmill at the time, what her secret was. She answered, "When you walk with God, you have purpose, so you live longer. And you have peace and a positive attitude, so you live better."

Faith can help your health in three different ways. First, people who rely on God often have a feeling that "someone else is watching out for me." They don't feel they're going it alone. Next, people of faith are more able to unburden themselves. They separate situations into a) things they can do something about, and b) things they can't do something about. They then give the latter to God to fix! And finally, people with faith who pray regularly are practicing a form of meditation. Studies at Stanford University and the University of North Carolina show that prayer works as well as meditation to help control stress and anxiety, and thereby protect your health.

It took me some time to rely on God as a partner in my efforts. At first I was simply frustrated and angry. I was young and in the midst of building a career, raising a family and contributing to my community. Moreover, I didn't beat my wife, steal from the poor or kick the family dog. Why had coronary heart disease struck me and threatened my life and family? I questioned God's intent. Then it occurred to me that when you can't figure it out, you need to faith it out, and I came to a place of peace.

From that point on, I had faith that with His help there would be a healthier future for my family and me. My faith grew into an understanding that even if I didn't know why this disaster had found me, it was a part of God's larger plan. My thinking changed from complaining about the past to praying and living for the future. I knew that I was not alone on my road to a healthy heart, and I looked to God for support and direction. I often thought of the timeless words of Margaret Fishback Powers:

One night I dreamed a dream.
I was walking along the beach with my Lord.
Across the dark sky flashed scenes from my life.
For each scene, I noticed two sets of footprints in the sand,
*   one belonging to me and one to my Lord.*

When the last scene of my life shot before me,
I looked back at the footprints in the sand.
There was only one set of footprints.
I realized that this was at the lowest and saddest time
*   of my life.*
This always bothered me and I questioned the Lord
*   about my dilemma.*

"Lord, You told me when I decided to follow You,
You would walk and talk with me all the way.
But I'm aware that during the most troublesome times
Of my life there is only one set of footprints.
I just don't understand why, when I needed You most,
You leave me."

He whispered, "My precious child,
I love you and will never leave you,
Never, ever, during your trials and testings.
When you saw only one set of footprints,
It was then that I carried you.

A Last Word

It's been said that health is not something to have but something to become. It's a process during which choices are made and, over time, habits are established. But that only happens if the change becomes part of who you are.

Everyone can benefit from inspiration on this journey. For me, the motivation came from my young family. I just had to look at them and I was moved to do the right thing. I also found that reading quotes, stories and anecdotes helped me along the way.

Here's the routine that helps me prepare mentally for managing my physical health: As soon as I wake up, I thank God for all that He has given me—my life, my family, my work and, in particular, this day. Then I look at the pictures of my family on our nightstand so that I understand why I want to be healthy. And finally, I read a story, quote or anecdote to help me think and act in a positive way.

However you use this material, remember that the key ingredient is *you*. Only you can start the process, only you can make the changes that will lead you to good health. Good health is yours for the choosing. You have to *want* it. In other words, you can't have tomorrow if you don't want today.

It *is* a choice. Why don't you make it?

PART TWO

The Motivations

DAY
1

My radio alarm clock, set as usual for 5:00 A.M. to wake me up for my morning run, went off on a cold, rainy Pacific Northwest day. I needed to get up but instead continued to lie snugly in bed, listening to the rain pelt my bedroom windows. After about 10 minutes of procrastination, I heard the radio announcer say something that got my attention. He related that the last finisher in the 1986 New York City Marathon—number 19,413—was a man named Bob Ireland. Bob, who was 40 years old, had his legs blown off in Vietnam. He became the first person to run a marathon with his arms instead of his legs, completing the course in 4 days, 2 hours, 48 minutes and 17 seconds.

Let's back up to the time after the alarm went off and before I learned about Bob. It felt so warm and cozy under my down comforter that I was seriously thinking about skipping my morning run. Then I heard the story of Bob's amazing feat. That was enough to get me to throw off the covers. But I got sort of "stuck" on the side of the bed and just sat there, motionless, listening to the downpour. Then I thought, *I have two good legs. How can I not use them?* By 5:30 I was laced up and out the door. Sometimes we need a reminder of what real perseverance is and of how many blessings we have.

DAY
2

"There are no gold medals for the 95-yard dash."

—MAX DE PREE, BUSINESS INNOVATOR AND AUTHOR OF
LEADERSHIP IS AN ART

The power of this short quote comes not only from its
message—go the whole distance, finish the job—but also
from the man who said it. Max De Pree embodied integrity.
He instituted an open-management style at Herman Miller,
the furniture company founded by his father. And at a time
when many companies treated workers as cogs in a machine,
he dared to encourage creativity, diversity and respect for
employees. Under his leadership, revenues rose from $230
to $743 million.

Think what *you* can do if you commit to change.

DAY
3

If you can't summon up the willpower to live healthfully
(maybe you hit a day when going to the gym or passing up
French fries seems too awful to contemplate), take some
time to think about your kids or your grandkids. They
need you to lead them by example. Raised on fast food,
television, cell phones and computer games, children today
are more sedentary, overweight and out of shape than
ever before. The number of seriously overweight children
has more than doubled in the last two decades, and more
of them have elevated cholesterol and type 2 diabetes.
Indeed, the Centers for Disease Control and Prevention
predicts that today's children may be the first generation of
Americans *not* to outlive their parents.

You have the power to turn their lives around. Parents
who work out regularly and who share daily physical
activities with their children—playing catch, taking a walk,
kicking a ball—are sending a clear message: In this family,
fitness and health matter. So if you hit a day when you can't
do it for yourself, do it for someone else.

DAY
4

"Let me tell you the secret that has led me to my goal.
My strength lies solely in my tenacity."

—LOUIS PASTEUR, CHEMIST

Louis Pasteur's work eventually led to cures for anthrax,
rabies and cholera, and his methodology became the basis
for modern biochemistry. His theories were not easily
proven; he suffered many setbacks. But Pasteur pushed
on. For me, this comment on tenacity is the bottom line for
healthy living: Never give in, never give up, continue moving
ahead. To succeed at anything, you must be determined to
turn your attitude and knowledge into action.

DAY
5

When *Sports Illustrated* reported on the 2002 performances and earnings of the top 10 professional golfers, Tiger Woods came in at number one with an average 18-hole score of 68.56 strokes. Sergio Garcia was number 10 with an average of 70.0 strokes. Less than 1.5 strokes per round separated the two golfers, but the difference in earnings was huge. Tiger earned nearly $7,000,000 that year; Sergio earned just over $2,400,000. By being slightly better—remember, we're talking only 1.44 strokes—Tiger earned an additional $4,600,000!

This story speaks to me about the power of small changes. Slight modifications in lifestyle habits can add up to a big change in your health. A minuscule difference today—extending your walk by 10 minutes, choosing an apple rather than a Danish—can make you feel better tomorrow. Add in slightly larger changes, like opting to reduce your stress with exercise rather than alcohol, and pretty soon you'll be adding years and vitality to your life. Remember, a healthy lifestyle is evolutionary, not revolutionary. The secret to success is to do a little bit more . . . every day.

DAY
6

"Seventy percent of success in life is showing up."

—WOODY ALLEN, FILMMAKER

DAY
7

I love sugar. And believe me, it's easy to love. Sugar is *everywhere*—the key ingredient in a huge number of food products, many of which taste great. (This may be why Americans eat and drink over 150 pounds of refined sugar a year, mostly in the form of high-fructose corn syrup.) But I can't let a sweet tooth dictate my dietary choices. Excessive sugar intake is linked to obesity, type 2 diabetes, elevated triglycerides and metabolic syndrome—all cardiac risk factors. That's why we have to take the time to read labels, particularly when we're about to chow down on some baked goods or chug back a supersized soda. Look at the grams per serving and remember this simple formula: 4 grams of sugar equals 1 teaspoon. So if the label on a regular can of soda says it contains 39 grams of sugar, you're about to drink the equivalent of almost *10 teaspoons* of sugar. That's more than *3 tablespoons*. Can't quite visualize that? Go—right now, don't wait—to your kitchen and pour three tablespoons of sugar into a bowl. Take a minute to just look at it. Enough said.

DAY
8

Back in the late 1970s, David Rabin, a noted professor of medicine at Vanderbilt University in Nashville, was diagnosed with Lou Gehrig's disease. He was 46 at the time. Before long, he couldn't speak or write; the idea that he might continue to practice medicine seemed foolhardy. But then he learned about a computer that could be operated by anyone, however physically challenged, who retained the functions of just one muscle group. David Rabin still had strength in one part of his body: his eyebrow! For the next four years, he used the computer to speak to his family, write papers and review manuscripts. He taught medical students, had a consulting practice, wrote a textbook on endocrinology and received a number of awards. And he did all this with the only things he could control: his spirit . . . and his eyebrow.

We all need heroes, people who do the right thing under any circumstance, and David Rabin is mine. He took what he had and used it to the best of his ability. Could anyone do more? When I'm feeling challenged (my legs are saying no to spin class, or a hot dog is whispering my name, or I'm so busy that I skip my relaxation routine), I think of David. His example puts me back on track.

DAY

9

"You are not obligated to win. You're obligated to keep trying to do the best you can every day."

—MARIAN WRIGHT EDELMAN, CHILDREN'S RIGHTS ACTIVIST

This quote is a perfect follow-up to yesterday's David Rabin story. It reminds me that good health is not just a goal; it's a process brought about by persistence, focus and commitment. Sometimes we focus on the wrong things— a damaged heart, say, or an arthritic hip—that conspire to sideline us. And too often we settle for the obvious: knowing what we can't do.

A woman in one of my seminars told me that she had type 2 diabetes and needed to lose weight, but both her knees were bad. She proceeded to tell me all the physical activities she couldn't do. No question about it—she knew what she couldn't do. I suggested that she focus on what she *could* do. She ended up using a stationary bike and joining a water aerobics class, both of which worked out well for her.

The takeaway? Focus on what you can do. You may not be able to do it all, but you can do something.

DAY
10

Did you ever notice how goals that are simply spoken are easier to ignore than ones that are written down? That's why it's important to write down your health goals—as an acknowledgment of your commitment. You can know more about your triglycerides than your cardiologist knows, but without a serious commitment to a lifetime of healthy habits, you will fail.

After my bypass surgery, my exercise program was hit-or-miss. Some days I'd have time, so I'd do it. Some days I wouldn't. But exercise was too important to my health to treat casually. I needed to make it a priority. The first thing I did was take my calendar and write at the top of every page: I will exercise this morning. It was a start, a mini contract with myself. But what really made a difference was marking out one hour every morning for a meeting with "Mr. Nike," scheduling the rest of my day around that inviolable appointment. Thanks to that written reminder, which I saw every time I opened my date book, my commitment to an exercise habit became real.

My advice to you? Start with a written contract with yourself.

DAY 11

I was reading the other day that there's some kind of scholarly dispute about who actually said, "The road to hell is paved with good intentions." Frankly, it doesn't matter to me who wrote it. What does matter? Going the other way on that road. Resolve to turn your intentions into action. How? Did you read yesterday's entry? *Write things down!*

DAY 12

"There is what I call a '212° attitude.' At 211°, water is hot. At 212°, it boils. And with boiling water comes steam. And with steam you can power a locomotive. One extra degree makes all the difference—in business and in life. It separates the good from the great."

—MAC ANDERSON, MOTIVATIONAL SPEAKER

"Only I can change my life. No one can do it for me."

—CAROL BURNETT, COMEDIAN AND ACTRESS

The week following my surgery, I was included in a group of 12 male bypass patients who were invited to return to the hospital to attend a class on healthy eating. I was the only patient who showed up. The other 11 sent their wives! These men, all of whom had just had their chests cracked open, did not think they were responsible for what they ate. Instead, they saddled their wives with that responsibility (and guilt). No one can assume responsibility for another's health. Not only is it unfair, but it doesn't work. It is your heart, your health—and your responsibility.

DAY
14

Basketball coach Jim Valvano was riddled with cancer when he gave a speech accepting the ESPY Arthur Ashe Courage and Humanitarian Award. "To me," he said, "there are three things we all should do every day. We should do these every day of our lives. Number one is laugh. You should laugh every day. Number two is think. You should spend some time in thought. And number three is, you should have your emotions moved to tears, could be happiness or joy. But think about it. If you laugh, you think and you cry, that's a full day. That's a heck of a day. You do that seven days a week, you're going to have something special." As he closed his speech, he announced the start of the Jimmy V Foundation for Cancer Research. Its motto: "Don't give up, don't ever give up!"

I have often read and reread Coach Valvano's words as I've laughed, thought and cried my way through heart disease. I remember coming home from the cardiologist's office the day before surgery. Bernie asked, "What did he say?" My response (which was true) was "Take two aspirins and call me in the morning." We laughed for a full 10 minutes! And I remember turning my brain upside down trying to figure out how to manage this dread disease. Then there were days when I simply cried, thinking, *What if all this lifestyle change doesn't work? Who will care for Bernie and the kids?*

But I also focused on Coach Valvano's last thoughts— "Don't give up. Don't ever give up"—and made them my

mantra. Saint Paul said, "I have fought a good fight, I have finished my course, I have kept the faith." And that is the example Coach Valvano set for me. I know that heart disease may win in the end, but if that happens, when it happens, I'll know that I held my own for more than 30 years. That's a victory.

DAY
15

Have you been brushing and flossing regularly? It might sound strange, but taking care of your mouth is one of the smartest ways to reduce cardiac risk. Major causes of coronary artery inflammation, which can trigger a heart attack, include smoking, chronic stress—and the dental bacteria associated with gum disease. So, by brushing thoroughly, flossing faithfully and getting a professional dental cleaning every six months, you'll be saving your teeth and quite possibly your heart. This is a classic example of how taking care of the small things pays off in big health dividends.

DAY
16

From 1983 to 1991, a 544-mile endurance race took place annually in Australia over the rugged terrain between Sydney and Melbourne. On the day of the inaugural race, the starting line was jammed with world-class runners decked out in state-of-the-art shoes and gear. Amidst the throng was 61-year-old farmer Cliff Young, wearing rubber boots and bib overalls. After some debate, the race officials decided to let him in; after all, he'd paid the entry fee. The usual strategy for surviving this race was to run about five hours, then rest, then run a few more hours, then stop to rest, eat and sleep, and so on. Since he had no endurance training, Cliff Young knew nothing of this. No one had even told him you needed to sleep! So he just set off and kept going, at a trot that became famous as the "Young shuffle." Cliff won the race—by two days!—and became a national hero.

I love this story because it's all about possibility. Cliff Young wasn't limited by a view of himself that said "You can't do this" or "You can't do it this way." He did it his way and he won. About six months after my bypass surgery, I entered a 10K race. Although I'd been running regularly as part of my rehabilitation program, the race officials wouldn't let me enter without a doctor's note. "Heart patients don't run in 10K races," my cardiologist said when I approached him. I replied, "I don't see myself as a heart patient running a race.

I'm a runner who happens to have heart disease." Persuaded by my outlook (if not my wisdom), he signed the note.

What's your attitude? Are you truly open to all the ways you can become fit?

DAY
17

"The need to live a balanced, healthier lifestyle is just plain logical, whether it is for prevention or rehabilitation. You don't have to be a rocket scientist to understand that the grease you sandblast from your oven and soak off your dishes isn't something you want in your arteries. You don't have to be a physiologist to understand that regular, moderate physical activity is preferable to no exercise. And you don't have to be a genius to figure out that setting fire to tobacco leaves and inhaling the smoke doesn't make a whole lot of sense."

—STEVE YARNALL, M.D., CARDIOLOGIST AND AUTHOR OF *BEYOND MEDICINE*

DAY
18

Today, focus on eating foods rich in fiber—particularly the soluble kind that will help reduce your cholesterol, both total and LDL (the "bad" cholesterol). Soluble fiber forms a gel in the digestive system that interferes with cholesterol absorption and helps you get the stuff out of your system. Most people know about the cholesterol-lowering ability of oatmeal and oat bran because they've seen the ads on TV. But many other foods are good sources of soluble fiber: barley, rice bran, lentils, peas, beans, fresh fruit and vegetables. I love them all and eat them every day.

DAY
19

"We are what we repeatedly do. Excellence, then, is not an act, but a habit."

—ARISTOTLE, PHILOSOPHER

Okay, we're talking about Aristotle, but I have to say he really nailed it with this one! Frankly, it took me a while to absorb the full meaning of his words; now they're a crucial element of my long-term strategy. Here's how it plays out: If you eat healthy and exercise regularly, you're creating a pattern of repetitions, and over time those repetitions become a habit, a matter of course. When I started cutting down on fat to reduce my cholesterol and lose weight, I had to think about ordering my lunchtime turkey sandwich on whole-wheat bread with lettuce, tomato and mustard but no mayonnaise or cheese. (This saved me about 20 grams of fat.) After a few weeks, the order became a habit; the mayo and Swiss, a nonissue.

DAY
20

High in the Italian Dolomites there's a popular inn. It's a good day's climb to the top of the mountain, but you can usually make it to the inn by lunchtime. And that's when you separate the men from the boys. Some amateur climbers, feeling the warmth of the fire and smelling the good cooking, tell their companions, "I'll just wait here while you go to the top. We'll join up for the hike back down." Comfortable and contented, they sit by the fire or play the piano and sing mountain-climbing songs. But around 3:30 in the afternoon the atmosphere changes; people turn to look up the mountain, hoping, perhaps, to see their friends reach the top.

I can easily imagine the sheepishness of the hikers who stay behind. I bet most of them are thinking, *If only I'd kept climbing!* Ever start an exercise program in January with a friend? You dropped out in February, but she stuck with it. Now it's June and, some 25 pounds lighter, she looks and feels terrific. What are you doing? Kicking yourself. *Why did I stop?* you wonder.

Don't stop! Keep on climbing the road to good health.

DAY
21

"What's the secret of success in making healthy lifestyle changes? In a word, *persistence*. Many people try for a while, but results come so slowly that they quit and go looking for something easier. What they don't realize is that, if they managed to hang on just a bit longer, they could have improved their health dramatically. Good health is a marathon, not a sprint. In other words, it's what you do over time that really counts. Don't worry about one particular point in the race where you might not have stayed the course. Just get back on track and keep going."

—BARRY A. FRANKLIN, PH.D., CARDIAC HEALTH EXPERT

DAY
22

Allow me to remind you of the sheer number of benefits that regular exercise can bring. It can strengthen your heart muscle, boost protective HDL cholesterol, protect the coronary arteries, reduce blood clotting, lower blood pressure, manage stress and help you lose weight (if you need to). So of course it helps reduce your risk of heart attack and stroke! Robert Butler, M.D., an expert on aging, says it so well: "If exercise could be packaged into a pill, it would be the single most widely prescribed and beneficial medicine in the nation." Think about it.

DAY
23

Jimmy Durante, one of the all-time great entertainers, was asked to do a show for World War II veterans. He said he was very busy, but he'd agree if he could do one short monologue and leave immediately afterwards. When the time came, Durante got onstage, went through the short monologue—and then kept on going. After 30 minutes he took a final bow and walked offstage. Someone stopped him and said, "I thought you had to go after a few minutes. What happened?" Durante answered, "You can see for yourself if you look at the front row." Sitting there were two veterans, each of whom had lost an arm in the war— one his right arm, the other his left. Together they were able to clap, and that's exactly what they were doing, loudly and cheerfully. Talk about a positive attitude!

DAY

24

"If you cannot do great things, then do small things in a great way."

—NAPOLEON HILL, AUTHOR

When I started my running program, I envisioned myself as one of the great marathoners of the day. It was my lofty intention to keep adding miles each week until I could run the full distance. That would show everyone that a cardiac patient could recover enough to run the most challenging of races. Well, it never happened. After completing a few 10K "fun runs," I realized that I was no marathoner. That kind of greatness did not lie in *my* future! So I decided to focus not on distance, but on the quality of the run itself. My commitment was to do the best I could, to give it my all, at whatever the distance—and to do it faithfully. It's been 30 years, and I'm still doing it.

DAY
25

Give yourself a fat-free mustache. There are so many good
reasons to drink milk. It's rich in vitamins (particularly
vitamin D, which is critical to heart health), minerals,
protein and, of course, calcium. But you must avoid milk
that has cholesterol-raising saturated fat—especially whole
(full-fat) milk, which contains a staggering 8 grams of fat
per 8 ounces. As for the "2%" in 2% milk, don't be fooled.
At almost 5 grams of fat per 8 ounces, it's practically full-fat.
One percent "light" milk is fine, but the best choice of all
is fat-free (also called nonfat or skim), which contains less
than half a gram of fat per 8 ounces.

**Giving good advice is a cinch, but getting people to follow it
is another matter. When we started to make healthy changes
at home, my children, six and four, were happy to eat more
fruits and vegetables. (We were lucky.) However, they refused
to drink "blue" (fat-free) milk. My crafty solution? I mixed
what they were drinking (2% milk) with what we wanted
them to drink (fat-free), gradually increasing the fat-free
portion until it was 100%. But we always served it in the 2%
container. One day at breakfast my daughter asked, "Is this
milk any good?" "Tastes great to me," I said. "Why?" She
replied, "Because the label says it's a year old!" She'd caught
us out, but by then her taste buds had changed. If you have
trouble introducing lower-fat food into your diet, try tricking
yourself by gradually making it part of every meal.**

DAY 26

The stress of modern life can cause all kinds of problems, and it often keeps us from eating well and being physically active. Why are we all so perpetually stressed? Current research suggests that many of us are not living in sync with our core values and goals. Here's a way to check whether that's true of you. Write your own epitaph. If you were to die today, what would go on the headstone *based on the way you're presently living*? If you're a workaholic who doesn't spend much time with your family, you may end up writing, "Here lies the best marketing consultant on the west coast." Is that really how you want to be remembered? Maybe you'd rather have written, "Here lies a great parent and a wonderful spouse." If so, your way of life is inconsistent with your true values, priorities and goals. Work on putting balance back in your life.

DAY
27

There's a Chinese festival called Qing Ming, during which people express their grief for relatives who have died by grooming their graves and taking walks of remembrance in the countryside. According to legend, this custom began when a youth's rude and foolish behavior resulted in the death of his mother. He decided that he would visit her grave every year to remember what she had done for him. Sadly, it was only after her death that he appreciated her.

It is so easy to take what we have for granted, only to realize its value once it's gone. We do it with people and we do it with our health. I remember hearing about a man who didn't have time for exercise on Monday, had a heart attack on Tuesday and realized on Wednesday that he would have no trouble fitting exercise into his schedule. He was one of the lucky ones. I'm urging you: Don't wait until your health is threatened. If you're fortunate enough to have good health, do all that you can to protect it. It's a lot more fun to exercise for prevention than for rehabilitation.

DAY
28

"Before everything else, getting ready is the secret of success."

—HENRY FORD, AUTOMOBILE MANUFACTURER

I admit it, I'm a "ready, shoot, aim" kind of guy. But I've learned that it's much easier to adopt a healthier lifestyle if you take the time to prepare. (Abraham Lincoln summed it up perfectly. "Give me six hours to fell a tree," he once said, "and I will spend the first four sharpening the ax.") So, if you're serious about skipping chips and ice cream in favor of fruits and vegetables, then you should toss the junk and stock your refrigerator with the good stuff. Otherwise, when hunger hits, you'll devour the foods that you're trying to avoid. Be prepared.

DAY
29

"The future conditions you, not the past. What you commit yourself to become determines what you are—more than anything that ever happened to you yesterday."

—TONY CAMPOLO, PASTOR AND AUTHOR

DAY
30

Making a commitment to a healthy lifestyle can change you fundamentally. Think of caterpillars and butterflies. Caterpillars aren't very pretty, but once they break free from their "prison" and become butterflies, what was once ugly is now beautiful. Of course, the transformation involves struggle, but a creature that could only crawl can soar. The butterfly has a new capacity for life . . . and so can you.

DAY
31

An elderly couple were having an intimate dinner to celebrate their 50th anniversary. "What do you think has been the secret to our success?" the husband asked. "I'll show you," said his wife. She disappeared into the bedroom and returned with a shoe box she had always kept hidden under the bed. Looking inside it, the husband found two crocheted dolls and $50,000 in cash. "Years ago," his wife explained, "my mother told me that the secret to a happy marriage is never to argue. When I got angry, she said, I was to keep quiet and channel that anger into crocheting a doll." The man was delighted; she'd been mad at him just twice in 50 years! "That explains the dolls," he said, "but what about the $50,000?" "Oh," she replied, smiling, "that's from selling dolls!"

—AUTHOR UNKNOWN

Anger, rage, hostility—these are destructive emotions for anyone. But if you have underlying cardiac disease, they dramatically increase your risk for a heart attack. Indeed, anger ranks right up there with cholesterol and coronary inflammation as a cardiac risk factor. Researchers at Harvard have discovered that people at risk of a heart attack are two to three times more susceptible after an angry episode. In addition, chronic anger can keep you from doing what's required—exercising, eating well, not smoking. So don't rage, and don't stew. Instead, channel that energy you're wasting into changing your habits—and if you can figure out a way to make money at the same time, so much the better!

DAY
32

"Challenges are what make life interesting; overcoming them is what makes life meaningful."

—JOSHUA J. MARINE, WRITER

33

"You may be disappointed if you fail, but you are doomed if you don't try."

—BEVERLY SILLS, OPERA SINGER

Twice, General Douglas MacArthur was refused admission to West Point. But he was accepted on the third try and would march into the history books. Rudyard Kipling received a rejection letter from the *San Francisco Examiner* saying, "Sorry, Mr. Kipling, but you just don't know how to use the English language." Enrico Caruso's music teacher told him he had no voice at all and couldn't sing. Einstein's schoolteachers described him as "mentally slow, unsociable and adrift in his foolish dreams." By age 46, Beethoven was completely deaf, and he wrote five of his greatest symphonies without hearing a note. At age 66, after several political defeats, Winston Churchill became one of Britain's greatest prime ministers. You get my point, right? Life is about overcoming! So don't worry about failing; worry about not trying.

34

Here's a story I heard about Ty Cobb, one of the greatest baseball hitters of all time. He ran the bases with abandon, hit everything pitchers could throw at him and had a lifetime batting average of .366. Many years after his retirement, he was interviewed by a young reporter, who said, "You led the major leagues in batting a number of times, Mr. Cobb. But the players today are bigger and faster. If you played today, what would your batting average be?" Without hesitating, Cobb replied, "Around .298." "But, Mr. Cobb, you were the greatest hitter in the game. Why such a low average?" "Hell, sonny," said Cobb, "I'm 78 years old!"

Cobb was clearly playing with the reporter in his response, which is one of the reasons I love this story. Nothing breeds success like success. If you do something well today, you're more likely to do it just as well—or better—tomorrow.

POSITIVE MIND, HEALTHY HEART

DAY
35

"Once a man has made a commitment to a way of life, he puts the greatest strength in the world behind him. It's something we call 'heart power.' Once a man has made this commitment, nothing will stop him short of success."

—VINCE LOMBARDI, FOOTBALL COACH

DAY
36

"The will to persevere is often the difference between failure and success."

—DAVID SARNOFF, RADIO AND TELEVISION EXECUTIVE AND FOUNDER OF NBC

Ours is a hurried, harried life. We walk and talk fast; we even eat fast. And by bolting down our food, we find ourselves barely noticing what we've eaten and often eating way too much. That's a shame. The Mediterranean diet, by contrast, is one of the healthiest ways of eating in the world, not just because of the foods it incorporates, but because Italians, French, Spanish and other Mediterranean peoples take more time than we do to eat. They appreciate the simple act of sitting down to talk and eat with friends and family, and that allows them to get more enjoyment out of less food. A study that compared eating habits in France with those in the United States found that the average French person takes 22 minutes to eat a McDonald's burger and fries, compared with 14 minutes for the average American. Overall, the French spend more than 120 minutes a day eating, while we spend just 60. But only 12% of French people are obese, as compared with 34% of Americans.

DAY
38

"You don't get to choose how you're going to die, or when. You can decide how you're going to live now."

—JOAN BAEZ, FOLKSINGER

DAY
39

Let's talk turkey. Specifically ground turkey, which is often recommended as a low-fat alternative to hamburger. Did you know that the ground turkey sold in stores often includes fatty dark meat and skin, which means that 4 ounces may contain as much as 10 to 11 grams of fat? Ground turkey breast is a much better choice. Make sure the label says "skinless breast" and, just to be sure, check the nutrition facts. If it's truly skinless white meat, it should have no more than 1 to 1.5 grams of fat per serving.

How many times do we take the "virtuous" route only to find out that we're expending energy and thought on something that won't really help us at all? I can't emphasize enough the importance of simple knowledge. Read labels, find things out, don't take stuff for granted. You are the master of your destiny.

DAY
40

"He who deliberates too long before taking a step will spend his whole life on one leg."

—CHINESE SAYING

Okay, now let me contradict what I said yesterday, or at least modify it a little. It's true that you *should* collect information, seek advice and prepare for the changes you're planning, but you shouldn't get stuck focusing on the future. At some point, you'll actually have to start! As writer and evangelist Dawson Trotman observed, "The greatest amount of wasted time is the time not getting started." I know that the first line of any book I write is the hardest! So how can you help yourself? By coming up with a simple schedule. Set specific times for things you want to do and the things you're dreading. Each time you follow through, you'll feel better . . . and you'll find that achieving success comes more easily. Don't believe me? Try the scheduling trick if you're having trouble building an exercise habit. It works!

DAY
41

A wonderful television drama, *See How She Runs,* was based on the true story of a 40-year-old schoolteacher who, after being sedentary most of her life, began jogging to get into shape. She enjoyed it enough to enter the Boston Marathon even though she knew her time wouldn't be that good; her goal was simply to finish. The race turned out to be a grueling test of her body and spirit. She developed blisters; a bicycle ran into her. She kept on going. But within a few hundred yards of the finish, she fell, completely exhausted, unable to get up. Some of her friends strung a tape across the finish line and began to cheer her on. She lifted her head, saw the tape and realized her goal was within sight. She got up, took a few faltering steps and then, with a burst of energy, ran the final few yards, crossing the finish line as a winner.

The message in this moving story is that victory belongs to those who keep looking at the goal, not the going; not the process, but the prize.

DAY
42

"Life is 10% what happens to you and 90% how you respond to it."

—LOU HOLTZ, FOOTBALL COACH

I first read this quote at a time when I really needed it. I was just starting my recovery period at home, and I couldn't stop thinking, *Why me? What did I do to have this terrible situation thrust on me?* I kept playing out that awful week of diagnosis and surgery in my mind. But Coach Holtz's words made me stop and reorder my thoughts. I realized that the surgery and what caused it were nowhere near as important as my new life. The past was the past. It could not be changed; I had no control over it. But the future was all about my response to the surgery, and I had a great deal of control over that. The future was mine.

43

Give yourself the cushion of time. We are overscheduled. We work too hard. This is not good! Feeling perpetually pushed for time often leads to chronic stress (or, more accurately, distress). Stress can have a terrible impact on heart health. In addition to driving people to skip exercise, eat too much fast food or smoke, it can also cause elevated cholesterol, high blood pressure, blood clotting and arterial inflammation. Help yourself cope by expecting the unexpected; build that cushion into your day. Instead of cramming your schedule, fill it to 80%, leaving 20% for traffic jams, family illness and other surprises. And if there are no surprises, you can reward yourself with some time off!

DAY
44

A high school teacher stood in front of his class of 35 seniors. Before passing out the final exam, he said, "I know that since most of you are off to college next fall, grades are very important. Because I am confident that you know this material, I will give an automatic B to anyone who opts to skip the final exam." A number of students sighed with relief, jumped up and left the room. The teacher then handed out the exam to the students who remained. It consisted of two sentences: "Congratulations, you have just received an A in this class. Keep believing in yourself."

—AUTHOR UNKNOWN

I read this story a few times before daring to ask myself what I would have done. In my younger life, I may well have taken the easier road. But now I strive for a greater reward. Building a life based on healthy habits has been tough at times, but the reward has been incalculable—better health, a longer life, watching my children grow. No matter how hard and bumpy the road, I knew I could, and would, stay on it. I believe in myself. Try believing in yourself, too.

DAY
45

"Live each and every day as if it were your last—because one day you'll be right."

—Bob Moawad, motivational speaker

DAY
46

"I can't change the direction of the wind, but I can adjust my sails to always reach my destination."

—Jimmy Dean, businessman

I think Jimmy Dean must have been talking to my wife, Bernie, because his quote and her advice to me when I'd been moping along for two weeks after my surgery are so similar. As she said in the foreword to this book, you can't change the cards you were dealt, but you can change the way you play those cards. It's not the event that's important; it's how you respond to it.

DAY
47

If you're serious about losing weight, start out by keeping a food log. Record what you eat, how much you eat and how many calories that represents. (Go to the bookstore and buy yourself a calorie counter, or use one of the many online calorie counters.) That means *everything*: the half-slice of toast one of the kids left at breakfast, the handful of jelly beans from the receptionist's desk, the bite of dessert your friend offers you at lunch. And be sure to include salad dressings, coffee creamers and other easily overlooked foods. You can't adjust your diet if you don't know what your diet is!

Keep in mind that you need to lose 500 calories a day (3,500 per week) in order to lose a pound of fat. You can accomplish this by burning 500 calories in exercise (which is very hard unless you're a marathoner), by eating 500 fewer calories, or a combination of both approaches (the most realistic). Writing down your calorie intake will help you stay in control, particularly at the outset. As you get more educated about your choices, you'll be able to give up the food log. But not too soon!

48

A man walked into a bar and asked the bartender, "Do you have anything for hiccups?" The bartender slapped him across the face. "Hey! What's the idea?" said the man. The bartender smiled and said, "Well, you don't have hiccups anymore, do you?" "I never did," the man replied. "I just wanted something to cure my wife. She's out in the car."

—AUTHOR UNKNOWN

Make sure you have the total picture in mind when you develop a fitness plan. Don't make assumptions based on incomplete information. I know a woman who watches her diet so carefully that she never feels the need to exercise. But there is no magic in being a sedentary vegetarian. It's a mistake to assume that healthy eating offsets lack of exercise.

"The willingness to accept responsibility for one's own life is the source from which self-respect springs."

—JOAN DIDION, AUTHOR OF *THE YEAR OF MAGICAL THINKING*

How often do we hear people blame someone or something else for their problems? How often do we do it ourselves? The government, business, the media—it's all their fault! But we are not victims if we take responsibility for our own lives. It's not McDonald's that makes us fat; it's not the fact that some TV special is on exactly at the time we planned to exercise that keeps us from the gym. We're responsible for the choices in life that affect our health. Remember, for every one person whose heart disease originates with bad genes, there are 449 who have created their problem with a knife, a fork and an unhealthy love affair with their couch.

50

All physical activity is good for your health, but aerobic exercise is the best way to condition your heart. (You may even lose some weight in the process.) And research shows that aerobic exercise is most effective when done at a sustained moderate-to-vigorous pace. Assess your pace by taking the "talk test." If you can carry on a conversation with a fellow exerciser while walking briskly (or jogging, cycling, jumping rope, rowing, swimming, stair-climbing, using an elliptical exercise machine or dancing), you're most likely doing it right. If you can't exercise and carry on a conversation at the same time, you're probably exercising too strenuously.

POSITIVE MIND, HEALTHY HEART

DAY
51

A child got his hand stuck in a valuable vase. Before resorting to breaking the vase, his father said, "Son, relax. Just open your hand and pull it out." The boy said, "I can't. If I do, I'll drop my penny." I think a lot of us are like him, so busy holding on to something of little value that we cannot realize—let alone accept—what God offers us. I've found faith and trust in God to be a vital part of changing from my old, unhealthy life to my new one.

Healing a heart is not just about healthy eating and exercise; it is also about accepting God's help with the recovery—even if we do not understand His plan for us. In the words of Lauretta Burns:

> *As children bring their broken toys*
> *with tears for us to mend,*
> *I brought my broken dreams to God*
> *because He is my friend.*
> *But then instead of leaving Him*
> *in peace to work alone,*
> *I hung around and tried to help*
> *with ways that were my own.*
> *At last I snatched them back and cried,*
> *"How can You be so slow?"*
> *"My child," He said, "what could I do?*
> *You never did let go."*

DAY
52

"The longer I live, the more I realize the impact of attitude on life. Attitude, to me, is far more important than facts. It is more important than the past, than education, than money, than circumstances, than failures, than successes, than what other people think or say or do. It is more important than appearance, giftedness or skill. It will make or break a company . . . a church . . . a home."

—CHARLES R. SWINDOLL, PASTOR AND AUTHOR OF *THE GRACE AWAKENING*

When we were newly married, Bernie and I moved from Tacoma to Chicago, where I had a new job. The move was fine for me because I went to work every day, but it was difficult for Bernie, who had given up her teaching job and had no friends or family in Chicago. One day she baked a pie and I had a piece at dinner. The next day, feeling a little down, Bernie started to nibble at the pie. Before she knew it, it was gone. She was so embarrassed that she baked another pie, ate one piece and, without letting on, served it to me for dinner that night. But she was also so angry with herself for feeling like a victim that she worked on her attitude, went over to the local school district and got herself a job as a substitute teacher. We all get to choose, every day, how we're going to approach life. Bernie's shift in outlook ultimately made our stay in Chicago a happy one.

P.S. She didn't tell me about the pie until 20 years later!

DAY
53

Want to live longer? Then get moving—and stay moving! We all know by now that regular exercise can enhance the quality of our lives by boosting energy, stamina and endurance, and by promoting weight control. But it can also help us live longer. A study of almost 17,000 Harvard alumni found that the active men in the group had 35% fewer heart attacks and lived about 2.5 years longer than their sedentary counterparts. Moreover, fit persons who suffered heart attacks were much more likely to survive. Instead of sailing in search of the Fountain of Youth, Ponce de Leon should have stayed on land and walked!

DAY
54

"Without discipline, there's no life at all."

—KATHARINE HEPBURN, ACTRESS

The wonderful Miss Kate is quite right. There would be no life, certainly no healthy lifestyle, without self-discipline. That's the necessary element to get you up early to walk. It's self-discipline that leads to repetition (walking every morning for a month), and repetition that leads to habits (walking mornings for the rest of your life).

DAY
55

Judge Alexander M. Saunders Jr. told a graduating class at the University of South Carolina that there are two kinds of people: those who will and those who might. "As responsibility is passed to your hands it will not do, as you live the rest of your life, to assume that someone else will bear the major burdens, that someone else will demonstrate the key convictions, that someone else will run for office, that someone else will take care of the poor, that someone else will visit the sick, protect civil rights, enforce law, preserve the culture, transmit value, maintain civilization and defend freedom. You must never forget that what you do not value will not be valued, that what you do not remember will not be remembered, that what you do not change will not be changed and what you do not do will not be done."

Sounds a lot like the difference between a "can do" and a "will do" attitude to me.

56

"Do not let what you cannot do interfere with what you can do."

—JOHN WOODEN, BASKETBALL COACH

Try to stay focused on what you can realistically accomplish. Not everyone can be in a triathlon, and that's okay. Zero in on what's right for you. If the best you can do at first is walk briskly for 15 minutes on the treadmill, make it your greatest 15-minute workout ever. And know that pretty soon you'll be doing your greatest 30-minute workout, your greatest 45-minute workout, your greatest . . .

DAY 57

Making an effort to eat fish at least twice a week, preferably oily fish such as salmon, is worthwhile. The oil is a great source of omega-3 fatty acids, which can reduce the risk of heart attack by lowering harmful LDL cholesterol and triglycerides, help prevent blood clots and contribute to the body's production of anti-inflammatory elements. If you're not a fish fan, consider that it takes only about 7.5 ounces a week to help cut the risk of dying from heart disease in half. Some non-fish sources of omega-3s include leafy green vegetables, nuts, flaxseeds, canola oil and tofu.

DAY 58

You have to know where you're going. Don't be like Alice when she asks the Cheshire Cat: "Would you please tell me which way I ought to go from here?" "That depends on where you want to get," the cat tells her. "I don't care much where," she says. "Then it doesn't matter which way you go," the cat replies.

"If I knew I'd live this long, I would have taken better care of myself."

—MICKEY MANTLE, BASEBALL PLAYER

As great a player as Mickey Mantle was, he couldn't reach his full potential because of injuries. He didn't train in the off-season; he didn't cut down on late-night parties during the regular season. All the men in his family had died young, and knowing that, he was somewhat fatalistic about his own health. But genetic history is not predestination. I have seen people offset bad genes with healthy lifestyles. And I have seen people offset good genes with poor choices. You can't do much about your genetic makeup, but you can do a lot about the way you live.

DAY
60

Did you know that your mind can be an invaluable tool for protecting your health? Here's a great way to use it. First, visualize a healthier you. Then spend a little time thinking about your present activity level and move on to reflect on how it would feel (and how it may have felt in the past) to be strong and flexible, to have endurance, to be physically confident. Next step? Take off your clothes and stand in front of a mirror. I know, I know . . . but try not to judge yourself or feel guilty! Simply use that mind of yours to make an assessment of where you are now. Are you carrying a few more pounds than you should? Have you lost muscle tone? Visualize yourself as you'd like to be: stronger, leaner, healthier.

By being honest with yourself now, you can galvanize yourself to make changes for a healthier future.

DAY
61

"People often say that motivation doesn't last. Well, neither does bathing—that's why we recommend it daily."

—ZIG ZIGLAR, MOTIVATIONAL SPEAKER AND AUTHOR OF *SEE YOU AT THE TOP*

It would be great if simply knowing how to live in a healthy way could make it happen. We'd be a nation of fit people! But it doesn't work that way. To move from *knowing* to *doing*, you need motivation. That's why every day I look for people's stories and sayings to inspire me and keep me on track.

A horse fell into a well. Since the old rancher who owned him had no way to get him out, he decided he'd have to bury him. He began shoveling dirt down onto the terrified animal. Then the horse pulled himself together. "Just shake it off and step on it," he decided. No matter how much dirt came raining down, the horse just kept shaking it off and stepping on it—until finally he stepped right out of the well.

This little story neatly illustrates a universal principle: Life will either bless you or bury you; the difference lies in having the right attitude. (And I love the fact that the horse is smarter than the rancher!)

DAY
63

"A strong, positive mental attitude will create more miracles than any wonder drug."

—PATRICIA NEAL, ACTRESS

Patricia Neal is well-known for her award-winning acting career, but her best performance came from real life. Tragedy struck her three times. Her infant son was severely injured in an accident. A daughter died of measles encephalitis. And at the age of 39 she suffered three massive strokes and was in a coma for 21 days, followed by years of struggle in rehabilitation. But she never quit. She returned to acting, which allowed her to support the Patricia Neal Rehabilitation Center, serving almost 20,000 inpatients and over 30,000 outpatients in Knoxville, Tennessee. Patricia Neal: the epitome of resiliency and perseverance.

DAY
64

When asked what he had learned after years of trying to invent a storage battery, Thomas Edison replied, "I have not failed. I've just found 10,000 ways that won't work." The road to any kind of change is bound to involve bumps and detours, so be ready for setbacks and try not to dwell on them as mistakes or failures. Take them for what they are: learning experiences. If at a party you eat too many high-fat, high-calorie foods, it doesn't mean you "blew it." It isn't the end of the world. Focus on your successes, not your failures. And remember what Scarlett O'Hara said: "Tomorrow is another day."

65

Although the Declaration of Independence provides for the pursuit of happiness, it does not guarantee that the pursuit will be successful. Research shows that happiness is a product of both nature and nurture. About 50% comes from genetic variables—meaning that some people are programmed to be happier than others. Another 10% comes from individual circumstances, and a whopping 40% is a result of behavior modification. In other words, happiness can be learned.

These statistics make total sense to me. As television host Hugh Downs once said, "A happy person is not a person in a certain set of circumstances, but rather a person with a certain set of attitudes." And that set of attitudes can create a positive set of circumstances. Take time each morning to tell yourself, "Today I choose to be happy."

DAY
66

"Perseverance is the hard work you do after you get tired of doing the hard work you already did."

—NEWT GINGRICH, CONGRESSMAN

DAY
67

If you have heart disease, one of your top priorities is stabilization; in other words, not getting any worse. Think about it—about how successful you would feel if you could halt the progression of your disease. How to accomplish this? By eating a low-fat diet and burning a minimum of 1,600 calories per week. And how to burn 1,600 calories? Walk about 15 miles a week. Can you find five hours a week for your health?

DAY
68

"To give anything less than your best is to sacrifice the gift."

—STEVE PREFONTAINE, TRACK STAR

Steve Prefontaine was one of the top runners of the '70s. His signature style was to go to the head of the pack early and run as fast as he could. There was no "pacing" for Steve. He just wore everyone else out. Not many of us have that level of talent, but we can all tap into the desire to do our best. Sometimes, after finishing a run when I know I've done my best, I feel as if I'm Steve Prefontaine breaking the tape—no matter what my time. Remember, champions come in many forms.

DAY
69

An old man and his granddaughter were sitting in rocking chairs outside a gas station, greeting visitors to their small town. One tourist asked, "What kind of a town is this?" The old man replied, "Well, what kind of a town are you from?" "One that is critical and negative," said the tourist. The old man said, "Really? That's just like this town." Then a family stopped to talk, and the father asked the old man, "Is this town a good place to live?" "Well," said the old man, "what about the town you're from?" The father said, "All the people there are very close to one another and always willing to lend a helping hand." The old man smiled and said, "You know, that's a lot like this town." A little while later, his granddaughter asked, "Grandpa, how come you told the first man this was a terrible town and the second man that it was a wonderful place to live?" The old man replied, "No matter where you go, you take your attitude with you. And that's what makes your experience terrible or wonderful."

—AUTHOR UNKNOWN

When I first started to change my eating habits, I felt very sorry for myself and pined for prime rib, sausage and cheeseburgers. I actually stopped looking forward to dinner. One night when we sat down to a delicious meal of linguine with red clam sauce, Bernie said to me, "Quit moping

around over a lost cheeseburger! Appreciate what you have
and that you're here to eat it. Get your mind right." Her
bracing words helped me shake off my negative attitude and
appreciate the pleasures of eating in a healthy way.

DAY
70

"The greatest discovery of my generation is that man can
alter his life simply by altering his attitude of mind."

—JAMES TRUSLOW ADAMS, HISTORIAN AND AUTHOR OF *THE EPIC OF
AMERICA*

Yogi Berra, meet James Truslow Adams.

DAY
71

Weight training should be a big part of your exercise program. Why? Because it builds and tones muscles, increases the ability of the body to burn fat and strengthens bones. And some studies show that it can increase metabolic rate by about 7%, helping the body to burn more calories even when at rest. Before starting to use weights (or any kind of exercise program), get your doctor's permission. Next, have a program drawn up specifically for you by a knowledgeable instructor who's certified by the American College of Sports Medicine, the American Council on Exercise or the National Strength and Conditioning Association. Make sure that the program is personalized to your goals, that it stresses form over the amount of weight you lift and that it covers every major muscle group, including arms, chest, back, legs and abdomen. To notice a real effect, you'll probably need to do two sessions a week of 8 to 10 different exercises.

DAY
72

In the 1996 Summer Olympics, Canadian sprinter Donovan Bailey ran the 100 meters in a record 9.84 seconds. Reviewing the video of his run, experts noticed to their amazement that Bailey accelerated consistently for the first 50 meters, then slowed down marginally and briefly but surprisingly picked up acceleration again as he crossed the finish line!

Even if we have no intention of ever running a 100-meter race, we can emulate Bailey's pace by increasing our commitment, particularly after we slow down. So what if we're growing older? That just means we have more time to devote to exercise. I know I want to be accelerating when I cross the finish line. Or, as the folks at Maxwell House Coffee used to say: "Good to the last drop." I want people to say that about me, too.

DAY
73

"You've got to be careful if you don't know where you're going because you might not get there."

—YOGI BERRA, BASEBALL PLAYER

DAY
74

People who have a Type A personality are five times more likely to suffer a heart attack than more relaxed Type Bs. Classic Type A individuals are hard-driving competitors, always trying to accomplish more and more in less and less time. Combative, relentless "doers," they plow through obstacles and live as if they're always on a deadline. They feel guilty about relaxing and tend to measure success in terms of numbers.

If that's you, don't despair. Instead, build yourself an exercise habit. Physical activity, which acts as a tranquilizer, has been shown to be particularly effective in stress management. It reduces stress hormones and stimulates the brain's production of endorphins, the chemicals that make you happy and contented.

My daughter and son grew up playing youth soccer. When my daughter was about 14, her team went to play in Germany and then the German teams came here to play. So we were hosts for a week to two 14-year-old German girls. During their time off, we planned to take them sightseeing. My wife wanted to show them Cannon Beach, Oregon, one of the most beautiful pieces of coastline in the world. It's a three-hour drive from our house in Washington State, and I had just one day to do it. As a typical Type A, I said to myself, "Forget three hours. I'll make it in less!" Busily breaking the land speed record, I was pulled over by the state police. "How long since your

last ticket?" the trooper asked. "About five years," I said as he wrote out the ticket. Now, a Type B personality would have been content just to limp into Cannon Beach at that point. Not me! Within 20 minutes, I was flagged down for a second speeding ticket.

DAY
75

"You will never find time for anything. If you want time, you must make it."

—CHARLES BUXTON, BRITISH POLITICIAN

DAY
76

"It is not because things are difficult that we do not dare; it is because we do not dare that they are difficult."

—SENECA, PHILOSOPHER AND STATESMAN

DAY
77

It takes courage to commit to healthy habits at any time, but particularly when you're feeling weak or vulnerable. And, of course, that's when you need your courage most.

Frank was 79 years old when I met him in a cardiac rehabilitation program. He had experienced two heart attacks before undergoing bypass surgery, and now he was apprehensive that exercise might trigger a third attack. Despite the reassurance and encouragement that the staff gave him, Frank was still not convinced. But he walked on the treadmill anyway. When I asked him how he'd managed to make himself do that, he replied, "I knew I needed to exercise, but I was still afraid. Then I remembered what General Omar Bradley said during World War II: 'Bravery is the capacity to perform properly, even when scared half to death.' I guess that's where I am."

DAY
78

Watch out for sodium; it can trigger high blood pressure and increase your risk of heart attack. That's why the American Heart Association recommends no more than 2,300 milligrams a day, or about a teaspoon of salt. The real culprit here is less likely to be the salt we use in cooking and at meals than the sodium that is ubiquitous in processed foods. So read the labels, and when you do, be on the lookout for baking soda, baking powder, celery salt, garlic salt, onion salt, kosher salt, rock salt, seasoned salt, sea salt, sodium ascorbate, sodium benzoate, sodium caseinate, sodium citrate, sodium erythorbate, sodium nitrate, monosodium glutamate (MSG), sodium bicarbonate, sodium propionate, sodium saccharin and sodium phosphate. A rose by any other name is still a rose . . . and the same holds true for salt!

DAY
79

Taking in less sodium is a great first step toward lowering your blood pressure. But don't stop there. New research shows that boosting your potassium level to 4,700 milligrams a day could cut your risk for hypertension by 10%. It's easy to add potassium to your diet since it's contained in a wide variety of foods, including bananas, sweet potatoes, beans, yogurt, tuna, squash, tomatoes, carrots, spinach, prunes, peaches, lean pork and low-fat milk.

DAY
80

"Oh, my friend, it's not what they take away from you that counts. It's what you do with what you have left."

—Vice President Hubert H. Humphrey Jr.

All of us can choose how we define ourselves. It's a matter of perspective. After my surgery, I could easily have seen myself as a heart patient with limitations. Instead, I chose to think of myself as a survivor, someone capable of building on what I had left, which in my case was my life itself.

81

The National Center for Health Statistics estimates that more than 34% of American adults are "obese" and 6% are "extremely obese." And shrewd marketers have taken this into account. Are you aware that today's size 8 in women's clothing was a size 10 in our mothers' and grandmothers' day? Designers know that women are more likely to spend money on a dress if it makes them feel slimmer than they really are. Forget style. Instead, remember that even 5 or 10 pounds of extra weight can undermine your cardiac health. An eight-year study of more than 115,000 women aged 30 to 55 revealed that those who were as little as 5% overweight were 30% more likely than their leaner counterparts to develop heart disease. That risk increased to 80% in those who were moderately overweight, while those who were obese were 300% more likely to develop heart disease. The same goes for men. We know that eating too much makes us fat, but our sedentary lifestyle is even more troubling. In the opinion of cardiac expert Dr. William Haskell, "The major culprit in weight gain is lack of physical activity."

DAY
82

Here's some nasty news. You'll burn fewer calories running a marathon than you'll consume in a large hot fudge sundae. But not to worry; there's some good news to go along. The more physically active you are, the more your metabolism speeds up. And then you burn more calories, even when you're sleeping. An easy way to give your metabolism a boost is to vary the intensity of your exercise. Instead of walking at a steady pace for 45 minutes, walk for 10 minutes at your normal pace, then walk or jog at a faster rate for the next 5 minutes. Continue alternating for 30 minutes more. What you're doing is called interval training, and it's been shown to speed up metabolism and burn more calories than exercising at a more measured rate.

DAY
83

"Failure will never overtake me if my determination to succeed is strong enough."

—OG MANDINO, AUTHOR OF *THE GREATEST SALESMAN IN THE WORLD*

DAY
84

New York's Ground Zero is, as I write this, still a massive canyon—a stark reminder of the 3,000 people who died where the twin towers of the World Trade Center once stood. But how did New Yorkers respond to this terrible catastrophe? With shock, sadness and grief, yes. But also with the compassion and spirit of renewal found in Yakov Smirnoff's mural at the site. It bears the inscription "The human spirit is not measured by the size of the act, but by the size of the heart."

The ability to succeed in life often comes down to a single choice: how you react to what has been done to you, in the past or currently. As Holocaust survivor Dr. Viktor Frankl wrote, "We who lived in concentration camps can remember the men who walked through the huts comforting others, giving away their last piece of bread. They may have been few in number, but they offer sufficient proof that everything can be taken from a man but one thing: the last of the human freedoms—to choose one's attitude in any given set of circumstances, to choose one's own way."

DAY
85

Take an after-work stress-busting break. Five minutes will do it. Start with some deep breaths, and focus on the present. When you feel relaxed, recall or picture something positive you did during your workday. Then imagine receiving an award for your good work, filling your mind with positive thoughts. Obsessing about things that didn't go well can make stress last all through your precious evening.

DAY
86

It's easy to procrastinate when it comes to making healthy changes. The first step in overcoming procrastination is to take responsibility for your life.

No matter how hard you wish, the tooth fairy isn't going to come while you're sleeping and replace your poor lifestyle habits with healthy ones. You need to do something! Don't be a procrastinator. Most of us have the information we need to eat well and exercise effectively. So start your healthy living program today . . . and then keep it up, one day at a time. What you do today will dictate many of your tomorrows.

DAY
87

In 1948, General Hoyt S. Vandenberg, the air force chief of staff, noticed that there was no one present at the funeral of an airman; that deeply disturbed him. After he spoke to his wife, Gladys, about his desire for each airman to be honored at his burial, she arranged for members of the officers' wives club to take turns attending the funeral services. In 1972, Julia Abrams, wife of the army chief of staff, founded a similar group called the Arlington Ladies. Ever since then, someone from the Arlington Ladies has honored each deceased soldier by attending his or her funeral at Arlington National Cemetery. General Vandenberg received much praise for what he did, but the real heroes are the generations of women who have shown up, without fail, for the families.

Thank goodness we don't have to wait to be buried to be honored by the people in our support systems. They count for so much. Maybe someone you know picks up a particularly tasty and healthy snack for you. Maybe someone else reminds you about that Wednesday night yoga class. Or maybe there's a coworker who encourages you to walk around the block with him rather than go for a cigarette break. I could not have kept my program going over the years without Bernie's active help and encouragement. She is my hero.

DAY
88

Alcohol can have great benefits if you drink in moderation. It raises your protective HDL cholesterol and lowers harmful LDL cholesterol, so a glass of wine with dinner is associated with a reduced risk of heart disease and stroke. And many alcoholic beverages, including red wine and beer, are rich in powerful antioxidants. Should everyone drink alcohol for heart health? No. But if you do drink alcohol, be sure to limit the amount to two drinks a day for men, one for women. Any more and you're likely to gain weight and be more susceptible to accidents, high blood pressure and liver disease.

My mother told me many times, "Joe, use moderation in all things." Right again, Mom!

"Courageous leadership simply means I've developed convictions that are stronger than my fears."

—JOHN MAXWELL, PH.D., LEADERSHIP EXPERT AND AUTHOR OF *TALENT IS NEVER ENOUGH WORKBOOK*

This comment from Maxwell speaks to the very real difficulty associated with making tough decisions. It is, for instance, not easy to stop smoking. It is not easy to cut back on desserts. It is not easy to breathe deeply and let the anger go. But if you have a goal, whether in business or in health, and you really believe that change is vital to your success, you'll find the courage to make the hard decision and follow through.

DAY

90

Trust in a higher power helps us make positive lifestyle changes. Whenever I was frustrated with my struggles to establish healthy eating and exercise habits, God always showed up and helped me keep going. This is a common thread throughout the Bible: When we really need Him, God shows up. The rest of the time, which is most of the time, we need to "keep treading and trusting." There is no magic carpet. To achieve anything worthwhile you have to walk it out in faith, step by challenging step.

DAY
91

"You've got to get up every morning with determination if you are going to go to bed with satisfaction."

—GEORGE LORIMER, EDITOR IN CHIEF, *THE SATURDAY EVENING POST*

I've taught myself to understand that a balanced life is multifaceted. It includes managing stress, eating in a healthy way and exercising regularly. So every morning I make a reasonable plan for each aspect and then use determination to carry it out. Will I use deep breathing today to manage stress? If so, when and where will I do it? Where will I eat a healthy lunch? What time will I go to the Y? Fitness doesn't just happen. It's the result of a plan and the determination to see it through. When my head hits the pillow, I want to feel satisfied not just with my efforts but also with my results.

DAY
92

A high school science teacher took a large-mouth jar and placed several large rocks in it. He asked the class, "Is it full?" The students replied unanimously, "Yes!" The teacher took a bucket of gravel and poured it into the jar. The gravel settled in the spaces between the rocks. He then asked the class, "Is it full?" "Yes!" came the eager reply. The teacher produced a large can of sand and proceeded to pour it into the jar. The sand filled up the small spaces in the gravel. For the third time, the teacher asked if the jar was full. Again the students answered, "Yes!" Finally the teacher brought out a pitcher of water and poured it into the jar. The water saturated the sand. Now the teacher asked the class, "What is the point of this demonstration?" One bright young fellow raised his hand and responded, "No matter how full your schedule is in life, you can always squeeze in more things." "No," replied the teacher. "The point is that unless you place the big rocks into the jar first, you will never get them in. The big rocks are the important things in your life . . . your family, your friends, your personal growth. If you fill your life with small things, like the gravel and sand in this demonstration, you will never have time for the important things."

—AUTHOR UNKNOWN

Look at the "big rocks" in your life. Confess—do they include daily exercise, eating healthy and managing stress?

DAY
93

A Chinese proverb says, "Blessed are they who laugh at themselves for they shall never cease to be entertained." Smart! As I said earlier, hostile people—those with high levels of cynicism, anger and aggression—are at a much higher risk of developing heart disease and other chronic illnesses than their more easygoing counterparts. You hear kids say it all the time: "Chill." Why not give it a try?

DAY
94

"Our greatest weakness lies in giving up. The most certain way to succeed is always to try just one more time."

—Thomas Edison, inventor

DAY

95

Type 2 diabetes, one of the fastest-growing health conditions in the United States, is largely preventable. More than 85% of type 2 diabetics have the disease because they're overweight. You can lower your risk of getting full-blown diabetes by at least 80% if you lose as little as 5% of your body weight and commit to 30 minutes of exercise every day.

DAY

96

"You have to accept whatever comes, and the only important thing is that you meet it with courage and with the best you have to give."

—ELEANOR ROOSEVELT, FIRST LADY AND HUMANITARIAN

DAY
97

A women's conference was so crowded that the staff brought in extra chairs. Everyone had a seat but felt cramped and unhappy. The guest speaker, evangelist Joni Eareckson Tada, was a quadriplegic, confined to a wheelchair. "I understand that some of you don't like the chair you're sitting in," she said. "Well, neither do I. But I have one thousand handicapped friends who would gladly trade places with you." The complaining stopped immediately.

This story puts it all in perspective for me. Is it difficult to rise early in the morning, face a driving rain and jog five miles? Of course. Is it sometimes frustrating to skip rich desserts, especially if others are eating them? You bet. Is it as difficult as being confined to a wheelchair? No way. Every day I thank God that I'm able to walk and jog, to exercise and to have the determination to eat healthy food.

DAY
98

"Be assured that you'll always have time for the things you put first."

—AUTHOR UNKNOWN

I was always someone who put the important things last! As a child, I saved the best food on my plate to eat at the end of the meal. As an adult, I'd run through the checklist of routine things to do in the office before getting to the really important ones. And it was the same with my health. I'd head to the gym or find a way to relax only after everything else was done. Often that meant I ran out of time and didn't get to exercise or relax. Finally, I figured out that it was a matter of establishing priorities. For me, healthy living had to come first, since everything else—my work, the welfare of my family—depended on it. From then on, I learned to structure my day around my good health regimen. There are side benefits, too. These days, I get my important work done and leave the routine tasks for a lazy day of catch-up. Healthy *and* productive—who can beat that?

DAY
99

Red meat is a good source of protein, iron and the B
vitamins; however, some cuts are high in fat (particularly
saturated fat) and calories. Cuts such as T-bone steak,
prime rib, New York strip, rib eye, rib roast, brisket, pork
spare ribs and lamb roast can have 20 to 30 grams of fat
per 3.5-ounce serving. And few people limit themselves
to such a small amount (about the size of a deck of cards
or a bar of soap). That's why you have to "go lean." Beef
cuts labeled *round* or *loin* are lower in fat. When you're
shopping for pork, lamb and veal, look for *loin* or *leg* cuts.
And try to think of the meat as a side dish—something that
accompanies your vegetable and salad, not vice versa.

DAY
100

Time to face up to it. You fudged your diet at dinner last night. You fudged the night before, too. Today the scale is up by half a pound. It's tempting to fudge again tonight—after all, you've gained only half a pound. Don't do it! Get back on track so the half a pound doesn't turn into a 3-, 5- or 10-pound gain.

I try to keep my eye on the long-term goals. It's fine to miss a day of exercise or to enjoy a piece of birthday cake, but be sure to limit these indulgences. I'm not embarrassed or ashamed that I enjoy giving myself a treat now and then, but I'm careful to get back to my regular routine before any real damage occurs. This way, I'm set to enjoy that now-and-then treat the next time the occasion arises.

DAY
101

"We are all capable of much more than we think we are."

—LAO-TZU, PHILOSOPHER

DAY
102

Worrying can wreak havoc on a healthy lifestyle, so let's think through the things that cause you concern. Some problems can be dealt with in a straightforward way. If you're always late for work, set your alarm clock 15 minutes earlier and be done with it. If you haven't been able to reach your elderly parent for a couple of hours, don't sit there fretting—call a neighbor. In other words, do what needs to be done so you aren't tempted to deviate from your good habits. Of course, some problems are out of your hands. If you're sitting in an airplane circling the airport while your important business meeting is going on below without you, you simply have to realize that there is absolutely nothing you can do about it. When you land, you can call, explain the situation, try to reschedule the meeting. It's annoying, it's inconvenient, but it's life. Make a conscious decision not to waste your time and energy fretting over things you can't control.

DAY
103

Yesterday we thought about everyday worries and concerns. But what about the real, big-time worries such as being laid off, going through a divorce or caring for a sick child? Such stressful events often drive people to comfort themselves by eating and drinking too much and giving up on the exercise that might be one of the few things to keep them sane. So be kind to yourself in ways that do not damage your health. Take a break and go for a walk. Relax in a hot bath. Listen to music or read a book. Go to a yoga class. If you do such things to care for yourself, you'll be in a better position to deal with the significant stressors that life can throw at you.

DAY
104

For many years, an ugly concrete Buddha sat in a Bangkok neighborhood, mostly unnoticed. Then, in 1957, a priest decided to take the old statue to his temple. In the moving process, the concrete shell cracked, revealing the world's largest chunk of sculptured gold, standing eight feet high and dating from the 13th century.

Everyone of us is like that statue. Our core is what's valuable. Sometimes it takes a health event—being diagnosed with high cholesterol or having a heart attack—to peel away our concrete shell. When we respond to the event by turning to healthy habits, we discover the gold we have inside.

DAY
105

"If a man does his best, what else is there?"

—General George Patton

DAY
106

A reminder: Establish those priorities. We all get 24 hours, or 1,440 minutes, or 86,400 seconds daily. Surely, out of all that time, you can find a mere 45 or 60 minutes to exercise and improve your health. Keep your focus. The main thing is to keep the main thing the main thing . . . and living healthy is the main thing!

DAY
107

There's a poignant story about a man who went into his wife's closet and picked up a beautifully wrapped package. "This isn't any ordinary package," he said to his friend as he unwrapped the box and showed him the beautiful silk scarf that was inside. "She got this the first time we went to New York, eight or nine years ago. She never put it on. She was saving it for a special occasion. Well, I guess this is it." He placed the gift box on the bed next to the other clothing he was taking to the funeral home. His wife had just died. He turned to his friend and said, "Never save something for a special occasion."

Every day in your life is a special occasion. Make the most of today. It will never come again.

108

Every morning a gazelle wakes up on the African plain and knows she has to run faster than the fastest lion or she will be killed. Every morning a lion wakes up and knows he must outrun the swiftest gazelle or he will starve to death. It matters not whether you're a lion or a gazelle. When the sun comes up, you'd better be ready to run.

That's a fable that all runners love! But it has wider applications. A friend of mine experienced some chest pain while walking uphill, had it checked out by his physician and found that he had major blockages. He was given two stents. "I'm thinking of getting into an exercise program and eating better," he told me. "But is it really necessary with the stents in place?" I told him that his situation could have three outcomes: "First, you could live healthier and have the blockages shrink. That's called coronary regression. Next, you could live healthier and have the blockages stabilize. If you never got any worse than you are today, that would be a huge success. Or you could live your present unhealthy lifestyle and have the blockages grow larger, perhaps ending in a heart attack. You're the gazelle and heart disease is the lion. If you want regression or stabilization, get running!"

DAY
109

Here's a good strategy from the Japanese island of Okinawa, which boasts a high concentration of centenarians. Leave the dinner table when you're *hara hachi bu*—"eight parts out of ten full."

DAY
110

"Do it. Do it right. Do it right now."

—SIGN ON THE WALL AT NASA HEADQUARTERS IN HOUSTON

DAY
111

"And in the end it's not the years in your life that count. It's the life in your years."

—ABRAHAM LINCOLN, 16TH PRESIDENT OF THE UNITED STATES

We all want a long life. But obsessing about the number of years distracts from the essential question: How many of those years are healthy ones? Two people may live to age 85, but while one of them spends the last 20 years of his life in a golf cart, the other can't get out of a wheelchair. Both have achieved longevity, but only one has maximized his health span. Which one do you want to be?

112

Avoid trans fats. When polyunsaturated oils are hardened through hydrogenation into a solid or semisolid food product (such as margarine or commercially baked goods), a chemical change takes place that produces trans fat, or trans fatty acids. Trans fat is even more harmful than saturated fat in causing "bad" LDL cholesterol to rise and "good" HDL cholesterol to fall. A recent study found that increasing trans fat in the diet led to a 29% rise in the risk of heart disease. The American Heart Association recommends that you consume less than 1% of your total calories from trans fat. So, if you eat 2,000 calories a day, no more than 20 calories should come from trans fat—that means less than 2 grams a day.

Watch out for "rounding down" on food labels. The Food and Drug Administration allows food products with less than 0.5 grams of trans fat per serving to claim zero grams of trans fat. But if you put a spread on your bread at each meal containing .49 grams of trans fat, that comes to almost 1.5 grams of trans fat—perilously close to the suggested maximum of 2 grams and certainly not the zero grams of trans fat that you thought you were getting. The tipoff is an ingredients list that contains "hydrogenated" oils or shortening. If it does, you may be getting more trans fat than you think.

DAY
113

Besides being a great painter and sculptor, Leonardo da Vinci was a genius inventor, scientist and mathematician. His notebooks were hundreds of years ahead of his time, anticipating helicopters, submarines and other modern inventions. Until the end of his life, he was driven by a desire to know more. You don't need the mind or talent of Leonardo to be teachable. You just need to be open, receptive, eager to learn.

114

Salutation to the Dawn

Look to this day!
For it is life,
The very life of life.
In its brief course
Lie all the verities
And realities of our existence:
The bliss of growth,
The glory of action,
The splendor of beauty.
For yesterday is but a dream,
And tomorrow is only a vision,
But today well-lived
Makes every yesterday a dream of happiness
And every tomorrow a vision of hope.
Look well, therefore, to this day!
Such is the Salutation to the Dawn.

—KALIDASA, SANSKRIT POET

DAY
115

"Life loves to be taken by the lapel and told, 'I am with you, kid. Let's go.'"

—MAYA ANGELOU, POET AND AUTHOR

A little exuberance goes a long way. Give it all you have in the Zumba class! Get in touch with your inner Julia Child and cook a new recipe with gusto! Laugh at your own Type A characteristics. If you're living a healthy life, you'll be better able to live it to the fullest.

DAY
116

Exercise will lift your spirits much more than a drink or candy bar. One study showed that after just 30 minutes on a treadmill, people scored 25% lower on anxiety tests. The conclusion: The more you exercise, the better you'll feel. And virtuous to boot!

DAY
117

"Obstacles don't have to stop you. If you run into a wall, don't turn around and give up. Figure out how to climb it, go through it or work around it."

—MICHAEL JORDAN, BASKETBALL PLAYER

Who could argue with the best basketball player of his generation? He didn't get to be great just because of talent. He listened to coaches, practiced diligently and, most important, always found a way to get the job done. As President Calvin Coolidge said, "Nothing in the world can take the place of persistence. Talent will not; nothing is more common than unsuccessful men with talent. Genius will not; unrewarded genius is almost a proverb. Education will not; the world is full of educated derelicts. Persistence and determination alone are omnipotent." Just ask Michael Jordan.

DAY
118

"The greatest thing about tomorrow is, I will be better than I am today. And that's how I look at my life. I will be better as a golfer, I will be better as a person, I will be better as a father, I will be a better husband, I will be better as a friend. That's the beauty of tomorrow. There is no such thing as a setback. The lessons I learn today I will apply tomorrow, and I will be better."

—TIGER WOODS, GOLFER

Tiger is doing his part. Are you doing yours?

DAY
119

Ever play with a rubber band? If so, you know that a rubber band can't work unless it's stretched. Think about the times when you've been most successful in life and what it took to achieve that success. Stretch yourself, consciously, and you'll be surprised at what you can do.

120

Soft drinks are the enemy. There is absolutely nothing to be said in their favor. Not only are they crammed with calories, but those calories are empty calories—they do absolutely nothing to fill you up. So? You keep on eating. A group of participants at Purdue University ate 450 calories worth of jelly beans every day for four weeks and 450 calories worth of soda every day for the next four weeks. On the days they ate jelly beans, the participants decreased their normal diet by about 450 calories. The calories from the jelly beans replaced those from other foods, so the total calories consumed stayed the same. But on the days they drank soda, they ate what they always ate *plus* the 450 calories from the soda. In other words, they consumed 450 more calories than usual. The conclusion: Liquid calories do not satisfy, making it easier to overeat and gain weight.

DAY
121

At age 80, the Roman scholar Cato started to study Greek. His students were amazed and asked why he would attempt to learn a new language at his age. Cato replied: "It's the earliest age I have left."

Cato knew the truth: Learning is a lifelong process, not just an event during our school years. It's never too late to start learning how to live a healthy life. As we age, it's important not only to keep at it, but also to do more in the time that we have. As Tom Landry said, "Today, you have 100% of your life left."

DAY
122

"You can't get much done in life if you only work on the days when you feel good."

—JERRY WEST, BASKETBALL PLAYER

DAY
123

A study conducted in 2009 suggests that people with low blood levels of vitamin D have an increased risk of heart attack. So get your vitamin D! Here's how:

- Eat more foods rich in vitamin D, such as fortified milk, fish (particularly salmon, tuna and sardines) and eggs.

- Give yourself 15 minutes of sun exposure without sunscreen a few times a week.

- Take a daily multivitamin with 500 international units (IUs) of vitamin D.

Your doctor may suggest that you take an additional vitamin D supplement. Go ahead—ask the professional.

DAY
124

A frail old man went to live with his son, daughter-in-law and four-year-old grandson. The old man's hands trembled, his eyesight was blurred and his step faltered. At dinner, it was hard for him to eat tidily—he dropped his food and spilled his drink. Irritated, the son and daughter-in-law moved him to a small table in the corner, where he ate alone out of a wooden bowl. The four-year-old watched all this in silence. One evening before supper, the father noticed his son playing with wood scraps on the floor. "What are you making?" he asked. The boy replied, "I'm making a little bowl for you and Mama to eat your food in when I grow up."

—AUTHOR UNKNOWN

Children don't miss a trick. Even when you think they're not paying attention, they listen, they see and they take it all in. That's how they learn. If they see us living with healthy habits, that becomes the model for their lives. Wise parents realize that the way they live every day creates the building blocks for their children's future.

DAY
125

"Ability is what you are capable of doing.
Motivation determines what you do.
Attitude determines how well you do it."

—LOU HOLTZ, FOOTBALL COACH

DAY
126

"You don't have to be great to start, but you have to
start to be great."

—ZIG ZIGLAR, MOTIVATIONAL SPEAKER

**Getting started is at least 50% of the process. Speaking for
myself, I can tell you that the work I do in the gym is never
as difficult as making myself get out the door.**

DAY
127

Ask your doctor to sign you up for an exercise stress test. Usually done on a treadmill or stationary bike, it's a great way to evaluate your heart's pumping ability. This test also enables your doctor to assess your heart recovery rate (how much the heartbeat slows after you have exercised to exhaustion and then recovered). Normally, your heart rate would drop between 15 and 25 beats a minute after you stop exercising. The risk of dying within six years is four times greater among people whose heart rate falls 12 beats or less at one minute after exercising. Talk about a wake-up call!

DAY
128

There was a very cautious man who never laughed or played;
He never risked, he never tried, he never sang or prayed.
And when one day he passed away, his insurance was denied;
For since he never really lived, they claimed he never died.

—AUTHOR UNKNOWN

**Bypass surgery certainly altered my perspective on life. Now
I try to see each day as a gift, one that I can honor by living
my life to the fullest. I was lucky to have survived my cardiac
experience, and I know that today could have been a day
without me. I celebrate the fact that it *isn't* by dedicating a
part of every single day to maintaining a healthy lifestyle.**

DAY
129

"If you have made mistakes, there is always another chance for you. You may have a fresh start any moment you choose, for this thing we call 'failure' is not the falling down, but the staying down."

—MARY PICKFORD, ACTRESS

It's not what life hands you that counts; it's what you do with it. As writer Merle Miller says, "Everyone has his burden. What counts is how you carry it."

130

A man smokes three packs of cigarettes a day for 40 years, then dies of lung cancer. His family sues the tobacco company. A woman crashes her car while driving drunk, then blames the bartender. Your kids are out of control, so you blame television violence, lack of discipline in school or the influence of their friends. Excuses—there are more than enough to go around. But while blaming others may make us feel better, it keeps us from facing the truth in the mirror.

Most of us have made choices that contribute to our chances of developing serious diseases and debilitating conditions such as heart disease, cancer, type 2 diabetes and obesity. What we have to do is stop passing the buck, get honest with ourselves and start changing our ways. As Winston Churchill said, "The price of greatness is responsibility."

131

"Anything in life that we don't accept will simply make trouble for us until we make peace with it."

—SHAKTI GAWAIN, AUTHOR OF *CREATIVE VISUALIZATION*

Early on after my surgery, I had great difficulty accepting that heart disease was part of who I am. When I looked at other heart patients, usually some three decades older than me, I couldn't relate and would go into denial. I'd run fast, climb mountains and do hundreds of push-ups in an attempt to distance myself from the disease and other patients. But nothing worked. No matter what I did, the disease was still there. Finally, an older cardiologist took pity on me and gave sage counsel: "Heart disease is a part of you, like your black hair or the color of your eyes. Accept it and learn to work with it instead of against it." And I have.

Bob Gass of Bob Gass Ministries tells this story. After losing a baseball game, cartoon character Charlie Brown pours out his heart to Lucy: "All my life I've dreamed of pitching in the major leagues, but I'll never make it." Lucy says, "You're thinking too far ahead, Charlie Brown. Set yourself more immediate goals. Start with the next inning, for example. When you go out to pitch, see if you can walk to the mound . . . without falling down."

I love Charlie Brown's belief in his team, that rag-tag bunch that loses every game. Each spring, Charlie knows in his heart that his team will finally prevail. That's the attitude I try to tap into every morning as I face the day. Maybe I didn't eat so well yesterday; maybe I skipped exercise. But just like Charlie, I see today as a fresh start. I know I can do it right if I focus on the challenge at hand. Success starts with one step.

133

"Medication is of course important, but do not conclude that a pill dissolving in your stomach is necessarily more powerful than a healing thought dissolving in your mind."

—NORMAN VINCENT PEALE, PASTOR AND AUTHOR OF *THE TOUGH-MINDED OPTIMIST*

Dr. Peale brought the connection between mind and body home to many millions of people. We'd do well to remember his teachings today. In a nutshell, if you see yourself as healthy and follow that thought with positive actions, you may no longer need to rely on the pills.

DAY
134

Eating and TV don't mix. Why? Because watching television takes your attention away from your food, and the less you notice what you're eating, the more you're likely to eat. Don't believe me? Participants in one study ate a 400-calorie lunch, some while watching TV, others without TV. The watchers ate significantly more cookies than those who were not watching and continued to eat more even when the TV was turned off.

DAY
135

The Tatar tribes of Central Asia used a particular curse against their enemies: "May you stay in one place forever."

If you don't work every day on improving your health, you may stay in the same place forever, too. Not a good fate.

DAY
136

How you choose to live doesn't just matter to you; your healthy lifestyle becomes a role model for your children and grandchildren. This was driven home to me one Saturday afternoon as I watched the New York Yankees play the Boston Red Sox on television with my four-year-old son, Joe. My mother-in-law came into the room and casually asked Joe, "How's the game going?" "Oh, Grandma," he exclaimed with great concern in his voice. "The Yankees have two, but the b*****ds have four!" I couldn't even make eye contact with my mother-in-law, and to her credit, nothing was ever said to me. But from that day on, I realized that everything I did and said had an impact on my children. Knowing that, one of the messages I make sure to deliver is to eat healthy and exercise faithfully.

DAY
137

Don't be afraid to exercise after a heart attack. Sure, your doctor has to check you out and give you the go-ahead, but don't let fear get in your way of recovery. Says my friend Dr. Barry Franklin, "People who have had heart attacks often assume that they'll have another one within a year. The fact is that today increasing numbers of heart patients are entering their seventies, eighties and nineties, often outliving their counterparts without heart disease. Such patients not only take good care of themselves; they develop the mind-set necessary to deal with the challenges of heart disease. There is considerable evidence that we get what we expect and attract what we fear. Invariably, those patients who not only survive but thrive believe they can achieve longevity and a high quality of life."

DAY
138

"Always remember that God is looking out for you. When things look bad, remind yourself that God is bigger than your problem. Don't get worked up about what may or may not happen tomorrow. God will help you deal with whatever hard things come up when the time comes."

—FULTON BUNTAIN, PASTOR

God has been my partner in this journey to good health. I'm never alone at the gym, in a restaurant or when I close my eyes to relax. I know He is there to help me do my best.

DAY
139

Endurance is only a word until you have to deal with real problems, like a life-threatening illness. That's when the notion of staying the course becomes your anchor in the storm, your compass in times of confusion and the head of steam that gets you up the next hill.

DAY
140

"Death isn't the greatest loss in life. The greatest loss is what dies inside us while we live."

—NORMAN COUSINS, AUTHOR OF *ANATOMY OF AN ILLNESS*

Hospitalized with an undiagnosed condition, one that confounded his doctors, Norman Cousins spent weeks laughing at Marx Brothers comedies. Along the way, he discovered that laughter aids the healing process. A passion for life kept Cousins from giving up. So be like him. Develop a passion for healthy living. Laugh your way to health.

DAY
141

Take a walk for your health. The Nurses' Health Study found that women who walk briskly for 30 to 60 minutes five days a week cut their risk of stroke by 50% and reduced their rate of heart disease by 35% to 40%. There's another benefit, too. Exercise expert Jack Wilmore, M.D., says, "If walking regularly changes your metabolism even slightly, so that you burn an extra 100 calories a day, that small change can add up to 10 pounds of weight loss a year."

DAY
142

Some studies show that dark chocolate (not milk chocolate) can promote cardiac health. So treat yourself to everyone's favorite treat. "But only in moderation," says Jeffrey Blumberg, Ph.D., a nutrition expert at Tufts University. "It's simply too rich in calories, sugar and fat to be considered a health food."

DAY
143

"You cannot control what happens to you, but you can control your attitude toward what happens to you, and in that, you will be mastering change rather than allowing it to master you."

—BRIAN TRACY, AUTHOR OF *THE PSYCHOLOGY OF SELLING*

I stayed away from restaurants the first two months after my surgery. I was having enough trouble learning to eat healthier at home without putting restaurant meals into the mix. It was very much a two-steps-forward, one-step-back kind of dance. But finally I felt secure enough to take Bernie out to eat. Feeling smug in my new-found knowledge, I skipped the prime rib in favor of salmon. But it was served swimming in butter sauce—and was no better for me than the prime rib! I felt terrible about my bad decision and thought I'd never get the hang of healthy eating. Then something switched on in my mind, and I realized that I could choose to feel like a loser or I could respond positively. I asked the waiter to take the salmon back to the kitchen and remove the butter sauce, which they were happy to do. Then I made a mental note of questions I needed to ask next time I went out to eat. A positive attitude had turned a potential setback into a learning experience . . . and the salmon wasn't bad, either!

DAY
144

In their book *Now, Discover Your Strengths,* authors Marcus Buckingham and Donald O. Clifton propose that each of us is capable of doing one thing better than the next 10,000 people. They call it our "strength zone," a personal talent that can be cultivated to produce a high level of success.

Commenting on this "strength zone" in his own book, *Talent Is Never Enough,* Dr. John Maxwell says that people should focus the majority of their time and effort on their strengths, not their weaknesses. He proposes that people generally can increase their ability in an area by about 2 points on a scale of 1 to 10. So if your natural talent as a jogger is 4, with hard work you might become a 6. But if your natural talent at walking is a 7, you have the potential to be a 9 or even a 10. From a practical standpoint, I find that people stick with an exercise program if they like what they're doing, and people tend to like what they're doing if they do it well. So figure out which activities and exercises are in your "strength zone" and stick with them.

DAY
145

"He who fears he shall suffer already suffers what he fears."
—MICHEL DE MONTAIGNE, FRENCH ESSAYIST

I had always been physically active, in an on-again, off-again way. But after my surgery I became convinced that I needed to do regular aerobic exercise. So I told my doctor I wanted to start running. He was against it. In those days it was thought that heart patients should rest more and that exertion could trigger a heart attack. Although I was convinced that running was the right thing to do, I was immobilized by fear. Finally, after about two months of rest, I'd had enough. I bought a pair of running shoes, started slowly, and every day went a little bit farther. At my next checkup all the biometric data looked great—weight, blood pressure, cholesterol—and my doctor was impressed. That night he called me at home to ask, "What brand of running shoes do you recommend?" Guess he overcame his fear, too!

DAY
146

If you need some encouragement today, take a look at the palm tree. In a storm, it will bend—sometimes all the way to the ground—but it will not break. When the storm is over, it straightens up again. It is the picture of resiliency.

Think of the horrors that people are able to survive. We are made to bend without breaking. God promises to give us "strength that endures the unendurable and spills over into joy."

DAY
147

"Having a positive mental attitude is asking how something can be done rather than saying it can't be done."

—Bo Bennett, businessman and author of *Year to Success*

A positive attitude will help you focus, while a negative one simply throws up roadblocks in your path. If you can train yourself to keep an optimistic outlook, the solutions will present themselves. And the use of the word *train* in the previous sentence was intentional. Optimism is a learned behavior . . . start studying it now!

DAY
148

Take time to stretch. Working on your flexibility may not be as flashy as aerobics or weight training, but it's an important part of a complete exercise program. By stretching major muscle groups, especially those involved in whatever exercise you're doing, you'll maintain your flexibility and protect yourself from injury. And it feels so good! Right now, try it: Take a deep breath, and on your exhale reach up to the sky. Instant stress relief . . .

DAY
149

"When we do face difficult times, we need to remember that circumstances don't make a person, they reveal a person."

—RICHARD CARLSON, AUTHOR OF *DON'T SWEAT THE SMALL STUFF*

DAY
150

I recently took my five-year-old grandson, Joey, to his T-ball game. Everyone on the team looked great in new hats and uniforms, but unfortunately their playing skills didn't match the look. After hitting the ball, one kid ran from home plate to third base. Another couldn't locate his position in right field. And all were concerned about the postgame snack. I had worked with Joey on swinging the bat and hitting the ball, which sets on a tee, but his application of my teaching was a little erratic. As he dug in for his at-bat, I positioned myself behind the backstop. Then he took a prodigious swing . . . and missed! He set himself again and took another big swing with the same result. I felt devastated for him. Then he looked back at me, smiled and said, "The next one is going to the moon."

What a beautiful example of optimism, positive thinking and belief in yourself. His missed swings were in the past and he just knew this next one would be great. And it was! He drove the ball into center field. By the time the fielders could react and throw the ball in (remember, they were five-year-olds, too), Joey had crossed home plate. He had knocked it to the moon, just like he knew he would.

DAY
151

In the 1994 Western Open, golfer Davis Love III called a one-stroke penalty on himself. After marking his ball on the green, he wasn't sure that he had replaced it in the right spot, so he gave himself an extra stroke. That one stroke caused him to miss the tournament cut, and he went home without earning any money. (If he had made the cut, even finishing last, he would have earned $2,000.) This was important because at year's end Love was $590 short in the winnings needed to automatically qualify for the 1995 Masters, one of golf's premier events. Fortunately, he qualified with a win the week before the Masters and went on to a second-place finish in that tournament. Later he was asked how he would have felt if he had missed it because of calling a penalty on himself. "The real question," he said, "is how I'd have felt if I hadn't and spent the rest of my life wondering if I'd cheated."

Davis Love III always plays to win, but he does it the right way. I remember this story when I'm tempted to take a shortcut on my morning jog or choose potato chips instead of fruit with my lunchtime sandwich. That's a form of cheating. And worse, it's cheating myself.

DAY
152

"Attitude is a little thing that makes a big difference."

—WINSTON CHURCHILL, PRIME MINISTER OF GREAT BRITAIN

DAY
153

"Great effort springs naturally from great attitude."

—PAT RILEY, BASKETBALL COACH

I hope you're inspired by yesterday's quote from Winston Churchill and today's from Pat Riley—quite a duo! Though they operated in different theaters, they both knew—and proved—that a positive attitude leads to great achievements.

DAY
154

Creating new eating habits demands patience. It can take between six weeks and six months. Why so long? Because we have a lot to unlearn. We go to the doctor or a registered dietitian with an eating problem that took years to develop and say, "Fix me! I've got an hour." Unfortunately, an affinity for doughnuts doesn't develop overnight, and it won't disappear overnight. There is no pill, prayer or principle that will instantly undo the damage of years of poor eating habits. It requires hard work and—did I mention this?—patience.

As a Type A personality, I'm usually in a hurry to get things done. But one thing I learned was that you can't hurry the creation of a healthy lifestyle. Developing healthy habits, once and for all, takes time and effort. It is an evolutionary, not a revolutionary, process. So slow down. Relax. Commit to taking small steps each day, and give yourself enough time for the new way of eating and exercising to become habitual. After a few months, it will have fallen into place and you'll find you're a new person.

DAY
155

The carpenter who was helping to restore an old farmhouse had had a rough day. A flat tire made him late, his electric saw quit and at the end of the day his truck refused to start. While the owner of the house drove him home, he sat in stony silence, but on arriving he asked the fellow to come meet his family. As they walked toward the house, the carpenter paused briefly at a small tree, touching the tips of the branches with both hands. Then, as he opened the front door, he underwent an amazing transformation. Smiling now, he hugged his two children and gave his wife a kiss. Afterwards, as he walked his visitor back to his car, he explained the tree. "That's my trouble tree," he said. "I can't help having troubles on the job, but they don't belong in the house with my wife and the children. So I just hang them on the tree every night when I come home. Then in the morning I pick them up again." He paused. "Funny thing is," he said, "when I come out in the morning to get them, there aren't nearly as many as I remember hanging up."

—AUTHOR UNKNOWN

We all face daily trials, but we can't allow them to consume us. Leave your work problems at work so that you can be the best for your family . . . and for yourself.

DAY
156

"When we are no longer able to change a situation,
we are challenged to change ourselves."

—VIKTOR FRANKL, HOLOCAUST SURVIVOR AND AUTHOR OF
    MAN'S SEARCH FOR MEANING

My situation at the time of bypass surgery was clear. I had
high cholesterol, was not in good shape and had established
heart disease. I couldn't change the situation, so I was forced
to change myself by creating better eating, exercise and
stress management habits. Interestingly, as I changed over
time, so did my situation. Today I have less heart disease
than I did in 1977.

Long thought to be a "man's disease," cardiovascular disease has now been unmasked as an equal-opportunity killer. More than 450,000 women die of it each year in the United States, more than from the next 14 causes of death combined. For most women (and men), the risk of a heart attack is greatest between 6:00 A.M. and noon. In the morning, your hormone levels and blood pressure rise, and your arteries are stiff—all factors that contribute to clot formation. More heart attacks happen on Monday than on other days of the week, possibly due to the stress of plunging back into work after a relaxing weekend.

If I take time on Sunday evening to prepare for Monday, I find that some of the stress evaporates. I make a written list of my priorities and think about how they will be accomplished, and I discard lower-priority items. Once I'm mentally prepared, I'm ready to face the morning.

P.S. My first priority for Monday, and almost every other day, is . . . exercise.

DAY
158

"Be not afraid of going slowly; be afraid of standing still."
—JAPANESE PROVERB

DAY
159

It's hard to stay focused on health, but you must. Try visualizing a magnifying glass that focuses the rays of the sun and sets paper on fire. Or a laser beam focusing light to the point that it can cut through steel. Nothing is as potent as a focused life.

When I realized it was impossible for me to change my diet overnight, I began to focus on breakfast only: oatmeal replaced sugary cereals, whole-grain toast replaced Danish pastry and muffins, fruit became a staple. After about two months of the "new breakfast," those habits were firmly in place. Only then did I tackle lunch. Select your personal targets carefully and then focus, focus, focus on hitting the bull's-eye.

DAY
160

"Talent is cheaper than table salt. What separates the talented individual from the successful one is a lot of hard work."

—STEPHEN KING, AUTHOR

DAY
161

Get a pet! Studies show that having a pet improves both physical and emotional well-being. A pet is a companion, an animal to love and take care of, and, in the case of a dog, a walking buddy that will get you out of your house and into the world. One study followed heart attack victims for a year after the event. In that time, 28% of the people who did not own pets died, as compared with just 6% of pet owners.

DAY
162

Born with a congenital eye condition, W. Page Pitt had
lost 97% of his eyesight by age five. But there was no quit
in him. He refused to attend a school for the blind and
instead enrolled in public school, where he played baseball
and football. Graduating from college with a stellar record,
he became an outstanding professor of journalism at
Marshall University in Huntington, West Virginia. One
day a student asked Pitt which he thought would be worse:
blindness, deafness or not having arms and legs. "None of
those things," he replied. "Lethargy, irresponsibility, lack
of ambition or desire—they are the real handicaps."

**I had flown all day, Seattle to New York, for a meeting with
my publisher the following morning. It was 7:00 P.M. and I
was on a treadmill in the hotel's exercise room, feeling sorry
for myself. Why couldn't I be like other people, out on the
town, enjoying fancy food and a cocktail? Then I thought of
Pitt and all that he had accomplished in the face of much
greater odds. I ran a little faster knowing that he and I were
on the same team.**

DAY

163

"The only disability in life is a bad attitude."

—SCOTT HAMILTON, CHAMPION FIGURE SKATER

In the 1980s, Scott Hamilton was on top of the world as a skater. He won four consecutive U.S. and world championships as well as Olympic gold in 1984, and was one of the most popular athletes on the planet. But in 1997 life got more difficult. He was diagnosed with testicular cancer and found himself in a battle for his life. Scott fought it with style, grace and a positive attitude, overcoming the cancer and returning to skating. He certainly walked the talk of this quote.

DAY
164

Just do it. Really! Committing to a healthy lifestyle takes more than simply announcing your strategy. You need to step up to the plate. Believe in yourself and your plan.

Call it the "sure enough" syndrome. Expect to fail and, sure enough, you will. Expect to succeed and, sure enough, you will. Personal breakthroughs begin with a change in thinking. See yourself as eating healthy, exercising regularly, not smoking and able to handle the stresses of life. Believing this, deep down, determines what you expect, and what you expect determines how you will act.

DAY
165

"Your living is determined not so much by what life brings to you as by the attitude you bring to life; not so much by what happens to you as by the way your mind looks at what happens."

—KAHLIL GIBRAN, POET

DAY
166

"You've removed most of the roadblocks to success when you know the difference between motion and direction."

—BILL COPELAND, AUTHOR OF *ASHES TO THE VISTULA*

I know a woman whose fitness regimen is all over the place. She's always trying the latest fad diet, signing up for the newest exercise class and buying the advice book du jour. Unfortunately, she has no follow-through and she hasn't yet figured out that activity does not equal productivity, that motion doesn't equal direction. She's like a ping-pong ball in a boxcar—bouncing off the walls but going nowhere. You need to know where you're going in order to get there.

DAY
167

If you're not a gym person, try walking. A brisk walk of 3 to 5 miles will burn about 340 calories for a 150-pound person. To see real results for heart health, you'll have to expend 500 calories or more a week. For the maximum benefit, you should be expending between 2,000 and 3,500 calories a week.

DAY
168

A letter was returned to the post office. On the envelope was written "He's dead." Inadvertently, the letter was sent to the same address again. This time it came back with a stronger message: "He's still dead!" We often do the same old thing, over and over again, expecting different results. In this case, practice doesn't make perfect; it makes permanent. The secret to getting different results is to do something new.

169

My son-in-law, an orthopedic surgeon, told me about a patient who came in for a new knee . . . at age 89. "I still hike and I'm still active," the man said, "but it would be so much easier for me with a good knee!" The operation was successful and the patient went home. He returned for the other knee when he was 93. "I'm still going," he said, "but I'm afraid at my age, if I stop, I won't get started again." He got his knee.

Talk about a positive attitude! At age 89, this man saw himself as an active person and was looking for ways to continue. And he knew instinctively a key principle of lifestyle success: Don't stop! Age and condition may cause you to alter your pace or move to a new form of exercise, but they are not excuses to give up activity altogether.

DAY
170

"I discovered I always have choices and sometimes it's only a choice of attitude."

—JUDITH M. KNOWLTON, AUTHOR OF *HIGHER POWERED: A NINETY DAY GUIDE TO SERENITY & SELF-ESTEEM*

DAY
171

"Paralyze resistance with persistence."

—WOODY HAYES, FOOTBALL COACH

Remember, drops of water—one by one—can wear down a stone.

Don't forget your fiber. A recent study of 13,000 middle-aged men from seven different countries suggested that fiber, rather than fat, determined how successful they were at managing weight. In fact, the leanest men got a whopping 40% of their calories from fat, far more than recommended, but they consumed 41 grams of fiber a day.

Shoot for 25 to 35 grams of fiber a day. The best sources of fiber are fruits, vegetables, beans, grains and nuts. Vegetables are particularly good—for those who eat them. Unfortunately, about 25% of adults do not consume even one serving a day of vegetables. And one-quarter of all vegetables eaten are, you've guessed it, French fries.

DAY
173

As Gandhi stepped aboard a train one day, one of his shoes slipped off and landed on the track. The train started to move, so he couldn't retrieve it. Instead, to the amazement of his companions, he calmly took off his other shoe and threw it back along the track to land by the first. Asked by a fellow passenger why he did so, Gandhi smiled. "The poor man who finds the shoes lying on the track," he replied, "will now have a pair he can use."

This story has nothing to do with healthy living, but I picked it because I just love Gandhi's creative thinking and willingness to turn a negative into a positive.

DAY
174

"Winning isn't everything, but wanting to win is."

—VINCE LOMBARDI, FOOTBALL COACH

The fact is, when it comes to protecting my health, I can't do everything perfectly, every day. There are times when my legs feel like concrete, when comfort food wins over veggies and when I'm feeling depressed and anxious. But I always come back to healthy habits, to wanting the best health for my heart.

DAY
175

Do whatever it takes to establish a healthy eating pattern. You're bound to slip up now and then, but always remember that success comes from persistence. Cicero practiced speaking before friends every day for 30 years to perfect his eloquence. Noah Webster labored 21 years on his *American Dictionary of the English Language*. And Ben Hogan was known to hit over 500 shots on the driving range to prepare for a tournament. When it comes to your health, are you willing to persevere?

DAY
176

Disciplined people don't need cheering crowds to feed their hunger for excellence. Jascha Heifetz, perhaps the greatest violinist of the 20th century, practiced four hours every day until his death at age 87. That's more than 100,000 hours of practice, punctuated by occasional public performances!

It's not what you do in public that demonstrates character; it's what you do when you're alone.

DAY
177

"When everything seems to be going against you, remember that the airplane takes off against the wind, not with it."

—HENRY FORD, AUTOMOBILE MANUFACTURER

DAY
178

Keep a record of your exercise. Positive feedback reinforces behavior, which is why keeping an exercise journal is so valuable. As you watch your minutes and miles build, you'll feel enormously satisfied. Start by writing down a goal for yourself so you can see it every day—perhaps it's walking 50 miles in a month. As you get closer to the goal, you'll feel a renewed commitment. When you reach it, reward yourself with theater tickets or a new pair of exercise shoes. Then create a new goal and go after it.

179

"It doesn't matter where you start; it just matters where you finish."

—AUTHOR UNKNOWN

It can be discouraging to know that you have so far to go to be fit or to reach your weight goal when others are already halfway there. But it doesn't matter where you start. Reaching your goal is what counts. Here's some encouragement: Steven Blair, M.D., at the Cooper Institute followed nearly 10,000 men over a 10-year period. He found that those who moved from being "unfit" to "fit" had a greater reduction in cardiac risk than those moving from "fit" to "highly fit." So, wherever you start, making an improvement will bring you benefits.

180

Excuses are nothing but exit signs, so don't bother putting the blame on something or someone else. Claiming that the solution is beyond your reach is just a temporary way of letting yourself off the hook. But remember, it's easier to move from failure to success than from excuses to success. So examine your excuses and eliminate them, one by one.

I write this one from firsthand experience! Even though I knew that my diet had to get healthier, I still ate dessert when I traveled. I told myself, *Travel is hard. You deserve a treat now and then.* But there were many more "nows" than "thens." Finally, after a physical exam that showed no weight or cholesterol improvement, I had to face facts. Travel was just an excuse for me to indulge myself.

DAY
181

"Yes, we can!"

—BARACK OBAMA, 44TH PRESIDENT OF THE UNITED STATES

I don't care if you voted for President Obama or not, you have to be impressed with his positive attitude. It fed a vision, a plan and a campaign that resulted in his presidency. And my message to you: "Yes, YOU can!"

DAY
182

Be wary of weight-loss gimmicks such as "spot reducing." Basing their claims on the false notion that it's possible to "burn off" fat from a particular part of the body, deceptive advertisers promise that you can take inches off your waist, thighs or buttocks without vigorous exercise or dieting—and in just minutes a day. Nonsense! If spot reducing worked, people who chew gum would have skinny faces.

183

I was finishing up a business meeting in Los Angeles and looking forward to going home. My three o'clock flight would get me there in time for a dinner we were hosting. Bernie had reminded me at least three times not to be late, but I got caught up in the meeting and it ran long. By then it was one-thirty and my chances of making the flight were slim. I drove like a maniac through freeway traffic. Heart beating and legs pumping, I ran through the airport and just made the flight. And then we sat there. After the plane finally took off, I spent the entire flight fretting. When we landed, I rushed from the gate to the parking garage. If I drove fast, I could make the party. I turned the key in my car, and nothing happened. The battery was dead!

Too many of us live on adrenaline. We subconsciously put ourselves in pressure situations because we enjoy the rush that comes with them. The plane was going to be late taking off anyway; my car wouldn't start no matter what I did. Those things were outside my control. But deciding to allow myself enough time and to accept things I couldn't change *were* in my control. How foolish to give up that power.

DAY
184

"There are only so many tomorrows."

—MICHAEL LANDON, ACTOR

These words resonate strongly with heart patients and should resonate with everyone. The trick is to live by them. It's ironic and tragic that Michael Landon died of pancreatic cancer just three months after being diagnosed with the disease.

DAY
185

Eat your beans. Beans, peas and other legumes help your heart because they're great sources of complex carbohydrates, fiber, folate, protein, phytochemicals and other nutrients, but contain little or no fat and no cholesterol. Their soluble fiber is particularly effective in lowering blood cholesterol. Did you think oatmeal did the trick? Well, it's good for you, all right, but a half-cup serving of kidney or lima beans has twice the soluble fiber of three-quarters of a cup of oat bran or oatmeal.

186

"Talent is overrated. Great performance comes down to one thing more than any other: deliberate practice."

—GEOFF COLVIN, AUTHOR OF *TALENT IS OVERRATED*

When my son turned five, I began coaching his soccer team and couldn't help noticing a huge disparity in talent among the young players. Some were well coordinated; others, not. But during my 10 years as their coach, it turned out that the best players weren't the ones with the most talent. They were the boys who had worked consistently and with vigor to get the most out of whatever talent they possessed. I learned more from those kids than they ever learned from me.

DAY
187

When my father was in his eighties, his routine included a long walk each morning. But because of progressive arthritis he switched to walking every other day. Did he rest on the days he didn't walk? No, he just changed his activity, riding an exercise bike for 10 minutes and then following a Jane Fonda workout video.

I'm so proud of my dad's stick-to-itiveness. His circumstances changed and so did his workouts, but his attitude never faltered. What a wonderful message and example for our family! Don't forget to send the first and be the latter for yours.

DAY
188

"The moment you resolve to take hold of life with all your might and . . . stand alone, firm in your purpose, whatever happens, you set in motion the divine inner forces . . . implanted in you for your own development. . . . No power on earth can hold you back from success."

—ORISON SWETT MARDEN, FOUNDER OF *SUCCESS* MAGAZINE

189

Try to eat nuts regularly, particularly walnuts and almonds, since they're a great source of heart-healthy omega-3 fatty acids, right up there with fish. In the Nurses' Health Study, women who ate more than 5 ounces of nuts a week had a 35% reduction in their heart attack risk, as compared with women who ate 1 ounce of nuts a week or none at all. The downside: Nuts are high in calories, as you can see from the counts below, so eat them in moderation.

- 10 peanuts: 50

- 10 medium cashews: 92

- 10 whole almonds: 77

- 10 walnut halves: 132

- 10 hazelnuts: 89

190

Remember when the Emergency Broadcast System started? How irritated you were when it interrupted your favorite television program for a whole 30 seconds? The problems that disrupt our lives are a little like those tests. They're unscheduled and usually unwelcome, and they always seem to come at the worst possible time. But unlike the test patterns on television, life's trials don't necessarily arrive for a reason, and they certainly don't disappear in 30 seconds.

Trials can make us feel helpless, but we have control over one vital aspect of these situations—the way we respond to them. True, you can't turn them off like TV, but you can keep them in perspective.

DAY
191

"When you change the way you look at things,
the things you look at change."

—MAX PLANCK, PHYSICIST

Planck may have been speaking about the observer effect, the scientific principle that observing an experiment affects its outcome. But his words make just as much sense for life. I know that for a fact from my own experience, which I have observed!

DAY
192

"It does not matter how slowly you go so long as
you do not stop."

—CONFUCIUS, PHILOSOPHER

I've been talking a lot about persistence, but Confucius pretty much said it all in one short sentence.

DAY
193

Rhonda Byrne's best-selling book *The Secret* proposes that the shortcut to anything you want in your life is to be and feel happy now. This attitude is said to invoke something called the law of attraction, as in "If you think of things that make you happy, happy things will be attracted to you."

Obviously I'm a firm believer in positive thinking and being happy, but as a means to action; in other words, I believe you need a positive attitude if you're going to do the things necessary to improve your heart health. But listen to me: Thinking happy thoughts will not prevent a heart attack! Attitude without action is a specious goal.

DAY
194

"I will persist until I succeed. Always will I take another step. If that is of no avail, I will take another, and yet another. In truth, one step at a time is not too difficult. I know that small attempts, repeated, will complete any undertaking."

—OG MANDINO, AUTHOR OF *THE GREATEST SALESMAN IN THE WORLD*

One foot in front of the other . . . never giving up . . . you know what to do.

DAY
195

Contemporary exercise guidelines recommend at least 30 minutes of moderate-intensity activities five or more days per week. These can include cleaning your home, taking the stairs instead of the elevator and parking your car at the far end of the lot. Moderate-intensity activities can be accumulated in short bouts of 10 minutes or longer, as long as they add up to 30 minutes or more.

- An alternative is at least 20 minutes of vigorous exercise four days per week. This includes brisk walking, jogging, exercise machines such as a stair-climber and exercise classes such as aerobic dance or spinning. Remember, 20 minutes is a minimum.

- And finally, whether you use moderate-intensity or vigorous exercise, the guidelines suggest resistance training and stretching on two or more days per week.

Need I remind you that there are *seven* days in the week? The Lord only rested on one.

196

Get the scoop on soy. At one point, it was thought that a diet rich in soy protein would lower LDL cholesterol and promote heart health; after all, look at all those folks in Asian countries who eat soy and have low rates of heart disease. Jumping on the bandwagon, the Food and Drug Administration proclaimed that just 25 grams of soy protein a day, "as part of a diet low in saturated fat and cholesterol," could reduce the risk of heart disease. New studies, however, show that soy only minimally reduces LDL cholesterol and has no effect on HDL cholesterol or triglycerides. In a reversal of position, the American Heart Association no longer recommends soy foods or supplements for reducing cholesterol. And those people in Asia? Turns out their good heart health is less about tofu, soy milk and soybeans and more about what those soy foods replaced: meat!

DAY
197

A man named Devon received a phone call from his mother letting him know that their elderly neighbor Pete had died. After his own father passed away, Devon had spent a lot of time with Pete. That's where I learned how to fish, how to nail a board and how to drive, he remembered. But over the years he had lost contact. After the funeral, Devon attended a small gathering at Pete's house. He sat at Pete's desk, as he had done hundreds of times as a child, and realized something was missing—a small gold box containing what Pete described as "the thing I value most." A few days later, a package arrived for Devon. It was the box! Inside was a note: "Upon my death, please forward this box and its contents to Devon." Carefully unlocking the box, Devon found a gold pocket watch engraved with these words: "Devon, Thanks for your time!—Pete."

—AUTHOR UNKNOWN

This story really speaks to me because I, too, have come to value time more than anything else in life. When the doctors predicted I would not live to be 40, my thoughts were not of money, houses or vacations, but of the time, the life I would miss with Bernie, our children and grandchildren. But as a result of living healthier, I've had my time with them. And, as it was for Pete, time is still the most valuable thing in my life. Take the time to think about your time.

DAY

198

Vary your daily routine to stay energized and happy. Try a new route to work, take yourself to a new restaurant in town, stop to watch kids playing in a park. And don't forget more ambitious and long-term activities such as learning a new skill or language, or planning a trip to a new and exciting place. The challenge, the sense of accomplishment, the activity itself will help to bolster a positive outlook.

DAY
199

You'll love this one: Get a massage! The hands-on
manipulation of muscles and other soft tissues that is
the essence of massage actually improves your physical,
emotional and mental well-being. Massage stimulates
circulation, prevents and relieves muscle cramps, and
helps with pain management. And it's a wonderful way
to manage chronic stress. It fosters peace of mind,
reduces anxiety and promotes a relaxed state of mental
alertness. Massage is to the human body what a tune-up
is to a car. How fortunate that something so helpful feels
like such a treat.

200

"What's courage but having faith instead of fear?"

—MICHAEL J. FOX, ACTOR

In 1964, President Eisenhower went to visit Winston Churchill. The former prime minister was dying and Eisenhower sat by his bed for a long time, remembering how Great Britain's bold-spirited leader had never lost faith in victory, even in the face of German air raids on his country. After a while, Churchill laboriously raised his hand and made the famous "V" for victory sign that he had so often flashed to the British people during the Battle of Britain. That sign was the physical embodiment of faith over fear. Eisenhower, fighting back tears, pushed his chair back, stood up, saluted him and left the room.

DAY
201

A salesman who always drove an old car and wore dingy clothes showed up one day at his office in a BMW and wearing a designer suit. "What happened?" his coworkers asked. "Remember how I used to worry about everything?" the salesman said. "Well, I hired a team of professional worriers; now I tell them my problems and they do all my worrying while I go out and sell." Asked how much they charge, he answered, "About $5,000 a week." Then, asked how he could afford that, he smiled and said, "That's their worry, not mine!"

—AUTHOR UNKNOWN

Wouldn't you like to have somebody to handle all your worries? Many people do. They hand them to God (who doesn't charge a cent). Think about it. Instead of wasting today fretting about tomorrow, you could get busy living the life He gave you to enjoy.

DAY
202

"The difference between the impossible and the possible lies in a man's determination."

—TOMMY LASORDA, BASEBALL MANAGER

DAY
203

Use healthier spreads. Try to avoid butter, which contains saturated fat, and stick margarine, which contains trans fat. Both can raise your LDL cholesterol. Choose liquid or soft margarine made from unsaturated fat, such as Smart Balance. Also, look for the newer types of margarine made with plant sterol esters, such as Benecol Spreads and Take Control's Promise and Supershots spreads; they can lower cholesterol the way oat bran does.

DAY
204

It was the top of the second inning in a softball game between Central Washington University and Western Oregon University. Central Washington was two games down in their series and needed a win to keep playoff hopes alive. Central was winning, 2–1, but with two on base diminutive Sara Tucholsky hit a home run for Western, her first ever. As she rounded first base, her knee buckled and she collapsed in pain. The two teams met with the umpire, who explained the rules: "No one on her team can touch her, or she's out. If she can't make it around the bases, she's also out." It was obvious that Sara couldn't make it. Then Mallory Holtman, who was playing first base for Central, spoke up. "Excuse me," she said, "but would it be okay if we carried her around and she touched each bag?" The officials huddled and said it would be legal. So Mallory and Liz Wallace, the Central shortstop, picked Sara up and carried her around the bases, helping her to touch each one and giving Western the edge and ultimately the win.

Winning can take a lot of different forms, but doing the right thing always makes you a winner.

DAY
205

The importance of diet, exercise and positive thinking in adding good years to your life cannot be overemphasized. But don't forget to socialize! Isolation and loneliness can be very destructive to your physical and mental health and can lead to depression, which often triggers heart attacks. You need the regular company of friends and family. Women generally have better support systems as they age than men do. This may be a factor in why women generally outlive men.

DAY
206

To cut down on the stress in your life, avoid committing to things you can't or don't want to do. Taking on too many responsibilities and failing is much more stressful than saying no to a request in the first place.

DAY
207

One morning, some company employees arrived at work to find a sign on the door. It read: "The person who has been hindering your growth in this company has passed away. Please come to the funeral in the large meeting room." Puzzled, people began filing in to pay their last respects, everyone wondering, *Who was this?* One by one, they looked into the coffin and saw a mirror, reflecting their faces as they peered inside. A sign next to the mirror read: "There is only one person who is capable of setting limits to your growth. It is YOU."

That's right. It's all up to you. You're the only person who can revolutionize your life, the only person who can influence your happiness, your progress, your success. Your life does not change when circumstances change. It changes when YOU change, when you go beyond the beliefs and habits that limit you and accept the fact that you are the only one responsible for your life.

DAY
208

"Nothing can stop the man with the right mental attitude from achieving his goal; nothing on earth can help the man with the wrong mental attitude."

—THOMAS JEFFERSON, THIRD PRESIDENT OF THE UNITED STATES

DAY
209

Listen to the specialists on this one. According to cardiologist Herbert Benson, M.D., the key to managing stress lies in learning how to produce a "relaxation response" to offset your "stress response." And since stress is endemic to our society, we must relax our mind and body on a regular basis.

Here's what that means in my language: Just relax! Every day! Take a walk, read a good book, listen to music, get a massage, soak in a warm bath. Or find something else that's particularly pleasant for you. Never use lack of time as an excuse. Make the time. Do it for yourself, because no one else will do it for you.

DAY
210

Wishing to encourage his progress on the piano, a mother took her young son to a Paderewski concert. Inside the hall, she spotted a friend in the audience and walked over to greet her. The little boy seized the opportunity to explore and somehow ended up on the stage. Suddenly, the curtains parted and spotlights focused on the impressive Steinway. There sat the little boy, innocently picking out "Twinkle, Twinkle, Little Star." Just then, the great piano master made his entrance, quickly moved to the piano and whispered in the boy's ear, "Don't quit. Keep playing." Leaning over, Paderewski reached down with his left hand and began filling in a bass part. Soon his right arm reached around to the other side of the child and he added a running obbligato. Together, the old master and the young novice transformed the situation into a gloriously creative experience. The audience was mesmerized.

—Author unknown

That's the way it is in life. What we can accomplish on our own is hardly noteworthy. We try our best, and the results may not be graceful, flowing music. But when we trust in the help of a Greater Power, our life's work can be beautiful. Next time you set out to accomplish something great, listen carefully. You can hear the voice of the Master whispering in your ear, "Don't quit. Keep playing."

DAY
211

Faith

*When you walk to the edge of all the light you have
and take the first step into the darkness of the unknown
you must believe that one of two things will happen:*

> *There will be something solid to stand upon
> or, you will be taught how to fly.*

—PATRICK OVERTON, AUTHOR OF *REBUILDING THE FRONT PORCH
OF AMERICA*

DAY
212

If you're tempted to skip the gym today, consider this:
Aerobic exercise will help you prolong your active life
and your independence. The typical aerobic power of a
60-year-old man is only 50% of what it was at age 20, so
it's harder to exercise without tiring. But researchers
have found that regular aerobic activities can help to
maintain lung function and improve the body's use of
oxygen by as much as 10 to 12 biological years.

DAY
213

The journalist Sydney J. Harris once wrote, "I walked with a friend to the newsstand the other night, and he bought a paper, thanking the owner politely. The owner, however, did not even acknowledge it. 'A sullen fellow, isn't he,' I commented as we walked away. 'Oh, he's that way every night,' said my friend. 'Then why do you continue being so polite to him?' I asked, and my friend replied, 'Why should I let him determine how I'm going to act?'"

Don't let the reactions of other people define you. When I first started jogging more than three decades ago, people weren't used to seeing grown men in shorts and running shoes on city streets. Did I look a bit strange? Yes, I did. But the looks I received never got in the way of my mission— creating better health.

DAY
214

"Life is like a game of cards. The hand that is dealt you represents determinism; the way you play it is free will."

—JAWAHARLAL NEHRU, PRIME MINISTER OF INDIA

DAY
215

"Problems are only opportunities in work clothes."

—HENRY J. KAISER, INDUSTRIALIST

DAY
216

Go for the healthy oils: olive and canola. Both are monounsaturated fats that help to lower cholesterol when you use them to replace saturated fats like butter or shortening. Olive oil adds a distinct flavor to food; canola oil adds no taste, so you can use it in baking.

You do need to remember that even these heart-healthy oils contain a lot of calories. So use them judiciously. As few as 50 extra calories a day—a little more than 1 teaspoon— can add up to 350 calories a week, or 18,250 in a year. That doesn't sound like much, but it equates to a gain of 5 pounds in a year or 52 pounds in a decade. Doesn't that low-fat balsamic dressing suddenly sound very yummy indeed?

217

Two nuns were on the way to the hospital where they worked when their car ran out of gas. They walked to the nearest service station, which didn't have a gas can. Then one of the nuns remembered that they had a bedpan in the trunk. They filled it at the gas station and carried it carefully back to the car. As they were pouring the gas from the bedpan into the car, two men happened to drive by in a big truck. Staring in disbelief, one said to the other, "Now that's what I call faith!" And were they ever surprised when those two nuns passed them on the freeway.

—AUTHOR UNKNOWN

No two ways about it, a healthy dose of faith helps you maintain healthy lifestyle habits. But the real lesson here is about flexibility—when things don't go your way, improvise. We all face roadblocks in life. They're part of the territory. You need to locate the ability that lies within you to respond creatively, whether that means going over, around or under the impediment. In other words, you need to keep moving. One evening I had a great dinner with friends at a nice restaurant. The dessert list was very enticing, and some of my friends indulged. I asked the waiter if they had fruit for dessert; he said no. "Do you have fruit as an appetizer?" I asked. He said they did. "Then I'll have an appetizer for dessert, please."

DAY
218

"Success is the sum of small efforts,
repeated day in and day out."

—ROBERT COLLIER, AUTHOR OF *THE SECRET OF THE AGES*

When I first started making healthy lifestyle changes, I
thought you had to do everything to the greatest degree
possible right away—run a marathon, become a vegetarian
and meditate daily. I gave myself two weeks to accomplish
these goals. Of course, I failed. Then I realized that a
different strategy might be more effective—small actions,
repeated daily. I made a commitment to eating two servings
of vegetables at dinner. It was a simple thing, but I did it
every day. Pretty soon, other healthy habits took hold: more
fish, less red meat; more complex carbohydrates, less fat;
portion control. Find one simple thing that you can do day
after day, put it in place and build upon it. It will be the
foundation for your new life.

DAY
219

Great news: Coffee is good for your heart! A 2008 study of more than 125,000 Americans found no connection between coffee consumption and increased risk of death. In fact, coffee drinking seems to be linked to a decreased risk of cardiovascular disease (especially in women), cancer and type 2 diabetes. That's because it's so rich in antioxidants. But if you're sensitive to the effects of caffeine, don't overindulge. You need that shut-eye.

DAY
220

"Don't waste mental energy brooding over past events or worrying about the future. Live a day at a time and do a job at a time."

—NORMAN VINCENT PEALE, PREACHER AND AUTHOR OF *THE POWER OF POSITIVE THINKING*

As we get older, it becomes easier to shrug off pointless worries. We tend to become more philosophical. If that describes you, take advantage of your hard-won knowledge. If that isn't you yet, strive to live in the moment. If you do, you may have more moments to live.

DAY
221

While browsing in an antique shop, a woman came upon a bag of coins. "What kinds of coins are these?" she asked. "Those aren't coins," said the owner. "They're Round Tuits. They're indispensable to getting things done." "I'll take them," said the woman. "For years my husband has been saying, 'I'll do it as soon as I get a Round Tuit.' Now he can accomplish all those things he put aside!"

—AUTHOR UNKNOWN

Ah, procrastination! It's the number one enemy of a healthy lifestyle. You can have all the information, set a goal and develop a "can do" attitude, but unless you act, all that is worth nothing. Too often it takes a frightening cardiac event—a heart attack or bypass surgery—to create the "teachable moment" that moves us to action. How much smarter to be preventive than to set yourself up for rehab.

DAY
222

"In recent years, scientific investigations have produced abundant information on the ways personal behavior affects health. This information can help us decide whether to smoke, when and how much to drink, how far to walk or climb stairs, whether to wear seat belts, and how or whether to engage in any other activity that might alter the risk of incurring disease or disability. For the two out of three adult Americans who do not smoke and do not drink excessively, one personal choice seems to influence long-term health prospects more than any other: what we eat. As the diseases of nutritional deficiency have diminished, they have been replaced by diseases of dietary excess and imbalance—problems that now rank among the leading causes of illness and death in the United States, touch the lives of most Americans, and generate substantial health care costs."

—C. Everett Koop, surgeon general

By eating the modern American diet, we're digging our graves with our forks. But you don't have to become a vegan (unless you want to) to be healthy. The Mediterranean diet is a wonderful model that balances health and delicious flavors. Remember, if the food doesn't taste good, no one will eat it, however healthy it is.

DAY
223

"Worrying is like a rocking chair; it gives you something to do, but it doesn't get you anywhere."

—AUTHOR UNKNOWN

DAY
224

The Bible says, "Do you not know that those who run in a race all run, but one receives the prize? Run in such a way that you may obtain it." Life is not a dress rehearsal. You only get to run once, so run to win. Make every lap count.

When you face a life-threatening situation such as bypass surgery, you come face-to-face with your own mortality and realize clearly that you have only one life, one chance to do your best. This is my thought every morning: to make the most out of today. And for me, that means honoring my commitment to healthy living, a race I'm still running to win for myself and my family.

DAY
225

Own your choices. How long are you going to tell yourself, *I know I need to change, and I will—tomorrow*? Sure, you have the right to consume chocolate cake and ice cream at bedtime every night. It's allowed, but it's not good for you, especially if you want unblocked arteries, healthy blood pressure, a trim waistline and the ability to exercise or at least keep up with your grandchildren.

Your character is the sum total of your everyday choices. Day by day, what you do is who you become.

DAY
226

"You must begin wherever you are."

—JACK BOLAND, CLERGYMAN

DAY
227

"You cannot plow a field by turning it over in your mind."

—AUTHOR UNKNOWN

I've made this point a few times, I know, but just keep reminding yourself to put your hopes into action. Think them through, mull them over . . . then make them real, tangible, something you can *feel*.

DAY
228

Stay hydrated. Most Americans drink soda, iced tea, coffee and sports drinks. But water—plain H_2O—hydrates the body better. And when you're hydrated, you're less likely to snack. When your brain receives the message that your body needs more water, that message may be interpreted as hunger, so you make a sandwich or down a bag of chips. Drink the recommended five to eight glasses of water a day and skip the snack.

DAY
229

"Do or do not. There is no 'try.'"

—YODA IN *STAR WARS: THE EMPIRE STRIKES BACK*

Take if from Yoda, one of the most renowned and powerful Jedi masters in galactic history, a legendary teacher. Achieving a goal, be it personal health or saving the Galactic Republic, is all about commitment. You either do it or you don't. There's no in-between.

230

A tourist visiting a small town asked an old man, "Can you tell me something this town is noted for?" After a moment's hesitation, the man replied, "Well, you can start here and go anywhere in the world that you want."

Nothing happens without a decision to start. Collecting information, buying a low-fat cookbook, installing a piece of exercise equipment—none of it's going to happen on its own. It's that difference between "can do" and "will do" that I've been trying to hammer home. This is the order: Make a decision, then act on it.

DAY
231

Today is the tomorrow I worried about yesterday,
And today was such a lovely day
That I wondered why I worried about today yesterday.
So today I am not going to worry about tomorrow.
There may not be a tomorrow anyway,
So today I am going to live as if there is no tomorrow
And I am going to forget about yesterday.

Today is the tomorrow I planned for yesterday
And nearly all my plans for today did not pan out
        the way I thought they would yesterday,
So today I am forgetting about tomorrow
        and I will plan for today
But not too strenuously.
Today I will stop to smell a rose.
I will tell a loved one how much I love her.
I will stop planning for tomorrow and plan to make
        today the best day of my life.

Today is the tomorrow I was afraid of yesterday
And today was nothing to be afraid of.
So today I will banish fear of the unknown.
I will embrace the unknown as a learning experience
        full of exciting opportunities.
Today, unlike yesterday, I will not fear tomorrow.

Today is the tomorrow I dreamed about yesterday,
And some of the dreams I dreamt about yesterday
came true today.
So today I am going to continue dreaming about tomorrow
And perhaps more of the dreams I dream today
will come true tomorrow.

Today is the tomorrow I set goals for yesterday
And I reached some of those goals today.
So today I am going to set slightly higher goals for
today and tomorrow
And if tomorrow turns out to be like today
I will certainly reach all of my goals one day!

—AUTHOR UNKNOWN

DAY
232

Be realistic. Set practical goals and expect to meet them.
Don't overload yourself with more work or commitments
than you can handle. That simply results in chronic
stress. Instead, let go of perfectionism. Your home doesn't
have to be spotless, and you don't always have to be the
last one to leave the office. And don't expect perfection
from others, either!

233

At the playground one day, a woman sat down next to a man on a bench. "That's my son over there," she said, pointing to a little boy in a red sweater who was gliding down the slide. "He's a fine-looking boy," the man said. "That's my daughter on the bike in the white dress." Then, looking at his watch, he called to his daughter. "What do you say we go, Melissa?" Melissa pleaded, "Just five more minutes, Dad. Okay?" The man nodded, and Melissa continued to ride her bike to her heart's content. Minutes passed, and the father stood and called again to his daughter: "Time to go now!" Again Melissa pleaded, "Five more minutes, Dad. Just five more minutes." When the man agreed, the woman next to him said, "My, you certainly are a patient father!" The man smiled and said, "Her older brother Tommy was killed by a drunk driver last year while he was riding his bike near here. I never spent much time with Tommy, and now I'd give anything for just five more minutes with him. I've vowed not to make the same mistake with Melissa. She thinks she has five more minutes to ride her bike. The truth is, I get five more minutes to watch her play."

—AUTHOR UNKNOWN

Life is all about making priorities, and often we don't fully appreciate our highest priorities until it's too late. While I liked to play sports, I didn't care for exercise before my surgery.

Taking a jog was a pain. Then came my surgery and, with it, a change in priorities. I remember being in bed, with multiple tubes in me, thinking, *What I wouldn't give for a nice jog in the park today.* What are *your* priorities?

DAY
234

"Anyone who has never made a mistake has never tried anything new."

—ALBERT EINSTEIN, PHYSICIST

My five-year-old grandson, Joey, was lobbying to take the training wheels off his bike. He did fine with the trainers but was now ready, he thought, for a new experience. I wasn't so sure. As he came down the long driveway, the bike picked up speed. He hit a pothole and fell off, scraping a knee. Not the least bit discouraged, he looked at me and said, "Forgot to brake. That won't happen again." He wasn't embarrassed or angry. His mistake was simply a learning experience. What a wonderful lesson for us grown-ups to remember.

235

Do you know the warning signs of a stroke? Call for emergency help if you or someone nearby suddenly experiences one or more of the following:

- Confusion; trouble speaking or understanding; slurred speech

- Numbness or weakness in the face or an arm or leg, especially if these occur on only one side of the body

- Vision trouble in one or both eyes; double vision

- Sudden unsteadiness; dizziness; loss of balance or coordination

- A severe, "thunderclap" headache or an unusual headache with no apparent cause

- Inability to stick out the tongue and move it from side to side

DAY
236

Reviewing his life, a man thought: *When I was young and free and my imagination had no limits, I dreamed of changing the world. As I grew older and wiser, I discovered the world would not change, so I shortened my sights somewhat and decided to change only my country. But it, too, seemed immovable. As I grew into my twilight years, in one last desperate attempt, I settled for changing only my family, those closest to me, but alas, they would have none of it. And now, as I lie on my deathbed, I suddenly realize: If I had only changed myself first, then, by example, I would have changed my family. And with their inspiration and encouragement, I could have bettered my country and, who knows, I might have even changed the world.*

—AUTHOR UNKNOWN

The politician Tip O'Neill once said, "All politics is local." It's the same with healthy living. Every positive change in our lives has to start with us.

237

"Never let the fear of striking out get in your way."

—BABE RUTH, BASEBALL PLAYER

Having struck out an amazing 1,330 times in his major league career, Babe Ruth might well have made baseball history as "the strikeout king" instead of "the home run king." But he didn't, because he never let a strikeout discourage him. He knew he would make up for it his next time at bat (he'd retire with 2,873 hits) and more than likely send the ball sailing into the stands.

To instill healthy lifestyle habits, we may have to make great changes. That's hard! We long for improvement but resist doing what's required. Being open to change is good, but we need to pursue it in an active way.

Dr. John C. Maxwell gets right to the heart of it: "Don't change your circumstances to improve your life—change yourself to improve your circumstances." I spent a lot of time moaning and groaning about my circumstances the first few weeks after surgery. "Why couldn't I have been genetically blessed with low cholesterol?" was a favorite— and particularly useless!—lament.

239

"Nothing will ever be attempted if all possible objections must first be overcome."

—SAMUEL JOHNSON, AUTHOR AND LEXICOGRAPHER

Don't wait until everything is perfect, because it never will be. Start from wherever you are and go forward. I remember starting to exercise with a friend. He was an experienced runner; I was a novice walker. When I voiced my concern that we weren't going at the same pace, he said, "I'm running five miles and you're walking two. But we do it in the same time. So we can start and end together. What could be better?"

DAY
240

A previous tip—call it part one—counseled that liquid calories do not fill us up. We eat the same amount of food as we normally would, so the liquid calories are just extra. Part two of my advice is to watch out for the amount of calories that we drink. They can be substantial. Most soft drinks, for example, contain more calories per ounce than are found in beer. And watch out for those fancy coffee drinks. A Grande (16-ounce) Starbucks Caramel Macchiato packs 240 calories and 4.5 grams of saturated fat. Grande, indeed!

DAY
241

The Incas told the story of a small bird named Tasoo who lived in the jungle. One hot summer day, terrible wildfires erupted and the flames devoured many trees and animals. Other birds flew high into the sky and far away to safety, but Tasoo couldn't bear to leave her precious jungle home to burn. Day and night, she flew with all her might to the river and back, filling her tiny beak with water to drop on the fires. Tasoo's rare courage and unshakable determination moved the gods to tears, and a great rain poured down upon the jungle, extinguishing the flames.

—AUTHOR UNKNOWN

Even the smallest actions of a determined spirit can change the world.

242

When my dad was in his early eighties (and in good health), he faced a quandary: to drive or not. He loved the freedom his car gave him, but he knew his reflexes were slowing down. God forbid he should cause an accident and hurt someone! One day I told him a study had shown that most auto accidents involving drivers seventy and older occurred during left-hand turns. Dad immediately got out a map and started plotting how he would get to his regular haunts while making only right-hand turns. He drove this way—making only right-hand turns—for the next two years. Then, at age 83, he turned in the keys.

My dad was the physical embodiment of the old (but true) adage: *Where there's a will, there's a way.* **Sometimes I wonder if a positive attitude might have a genetic component!**

DAY
243

Most of us have an overcrowded schedule from time to time, and looking at all the things that need to be done makes us feel anxious and overwhelmed. The trick is to tackle things one at a time, making certain to complete a specific task before moving on to the next. So review your schedule for the day or the week, then pick one item you need to get done or one decision that you can make fast—in five minutes or less. Once you've finished that, cross it off your list with a flourish and say out loud, "Done!" No matter how small the task, give yourself credit for doing it. Your sense of control and confidence will grow.

DAY
244

"Energy and persistence conquer all things."

—BENJAMIN FRANKLIN, STATESMAN, AUTHOR AND INVENTOR

To my mind, energy is a physical thing, but persistence is a mental decision. And of the two, I think persistence is the more important. A commitment to persistence will give you energy, but physical energy alone will not produce persistence.

DAY
245

"You may be on the right track, but if you just sit there you'll get run over."

—PAUL H. DUNN, LATTER-DAY SAINTS EXECUTIVE

Don't procrastinate. Take action to bring about success. Here's how to do it. First establish your goal, then back up and figure out what actions you must take to achieve it. Want to walk three miles in 45 minutes daily? Start by getting an okay from your doctor, then make sure you have a pair of good walking shoes and comfortable clothing, enlist a partner and start to walk. Begin with 15 minutes a day, then gradually add 5-minute increments. As you build up strength and stamina and speed, you will get closer and closer to your 45-minute, 3-mile goal until finally it's achieved.

DAY 246

"Knowing is not enough; we must apply. Willing is not enough; we must do."

—JOHANN WOLFGANG VON GOETHE, AUTHOR

It looks as if Goethe knew about the difference between "can do" and "will do" a couple of hundred years before I did.

DAY 247

Traditional snack foods—chips, crackers and candy— can pose a problem. Many contain trans fat and are high in calories. You can consume 100 calories, for instance, in less than half of a normal-size candy bar. A good tip is to make fruit your snack of choice. Look at all the fruit you can get for 100 calories:

1 apple, 5 apricots, 1 banana, ½ of a cantaloupe, 20 cherries, 1 grapefruit, 29 grapes, 1–2 oranges, 1 pear, 2 peaches, 1 nectarine, 2–3 tangerines, 3 plums, 2 cups of strawberries, 1 cup of raspberries, 10 ounces of watermelon or ⅕ of a honeydew melon

And no trans fat!

248

There's truth to the familiar saying "You are what you eat." And the same applies to the mind. You are what you think. Everything you allow into your mind, positively or negatively, affects your actions. And so do the people you associate with. Think of a positively charged person you know and how that person electrifies everyone else. Confidence is contagious.

Don't stay around negative, depressing people. Instead, try to fill your life with positive "will do" people. If you don't know anyone like that, immerse yourself in positive books, magazines and tapes, and eventually you'll find yourself attracting people of a like mind. It's always best to spend your time with the folks who inspire you.

DAY 249

"Nothing great was ever achieved without enthusiasm."

—RALPH WALDO EMERSON, ESSAYIST AND POET

Enter into living a heart-healthy lifestyle with enthusiasm. Relishing the small things—the smell of early morning air or the crunchy sweetness of a Granny Smith apple— can make it more pleasant to tackle the big ones.

DAY 250

Steer clear of fat-free baked goods, some of the real "bad guys" in the American obesity epidemic. Sure, the manufacturers take out the fat, but they often add more sugar to compensate and that jacks up the calories. (Your fat-free muffin could be 450 calories!) In addition, studies show that when we eat fat-free baked goods, we routinely consume three to five times as much as we normally would. So instead of eating a couple of regular chocolate-chip cookies (about 120 calories), we might gorge on 10 Fat Free Snackwells Devil's Food Cookie Cakes with 500 calories. Caveat emptor!

DAY
251

"In Chinese the word *crisis* contains two symbols: danger and opportunity. How do you choose to deal with crisis?"

—JIM MACLAREN, MOTIVATIONAL SPEAKER

Even events such as bypass surgery do not, of and by themselves, contain stress. When I went through bypass, was it a serious situation? Of course. Did I have great concern about the outcome? Most assuredly. But the event itself was inherently neutral. It was my reaction to the event that could produce stress. How we react to an event—that's what counts. What the Chinese are saying is that if you see the event as a crisis, your mind will interpret it as stressful. But if you view it as an opportunity, your mind will view it as a challenge. I chose to view the operation as an opportunity to "get well," a way to secure my future health. So, for me, concern never ended up as stress. It's all in how you look at it.

DAY
252

One evening, an old Cherokee decided to tell his grandson a story. He said, "My son, the battle inside us all is between two wolves. One is Evil. It is anger, envy, jealousy, sorrow, regret, greed, arrogance, self-pity, guilt, resentment, inferiority, lies, false pride, superiority and ego. The other is Good. It is joy, peace, love, hope, serenity, humility, kindness, benevolence, empathy, generosity, truth, faith and compassion." The grandson thought about it for a minute and then asked his grandfather, "Which wolf wins?" The old Cherokee replied, "The one you feed."

—AUTHOR UNKNOWN

For many of us, one wolf is complacency and indifference toward healthy habits and the other represents action and a positive outlook. Which wolf are you feeding?

DAY
253

"What you think, you become."

—THE BUDDHA

I made the same point only last week, I know, but we all need to come back to this thought time and again. The Buddha's words give me strength.

DAY
254

We've all heard that breakfast is the most important meal. It gets you ready for the workday; it helps prepare kids to learn in school. Now a study done at the University of Texas has reinforced that point regarding weight. The study showed that people who skip breakfast or have a poor breakfast end up eating more calories for the day. Breakfast is a meal where it's easy to eat healthy because of all the nutritious breakfast foods—whole-grain cereals and bread, fruit, eggs, milk and yogurt. But because of the morning rush that's part of our fast-paced lifestyle, or in an effort to lose weight by reducing caloric intake by one meal, many people skip breakfast. This is the worst thing to do. It seems that calories eaten earlier in the day provide a higher satiety level than those eaten later on. The Texas study found that participants who ate a healthy, reasonably sized breakfast of 400 to 500 calories consistently ate less throughout the rest of the day. When they ate no breakfast or one with just 200 calories, they tended to load up later. Bottom line: If you want to control your weight, eat a good breakfast.

As noted nutritionist Adelle Davis advised, "Eat breakfast like a king, lunch like a prince, and dinner like a pauper." Having a healthy breakfast is an essential lifestyle change that can bring about great results. Just making this commitment in the first place may be the most important breakfast change you make.

DAY
255

A 10-year-old boy decided to study judo, even though he had lost his left arm in a car accident. So he began taking lessons with an old Japanese master. After three months, the master had taught him only one move, saying, "This is the only move you'll ever need to know." Time passed, and the master took the boy to his first tournament, where he easily won his first two matches. The third match was more difficult, but after a while his opponent became impatient and charged; the boy deftly used his one move to win the match. Amazed to be in the finals, the boy was confronted by a bigger, stronger and more experienced opponent. At first, the boy appeared to be overmatched, but his opponent made a critical mistake. He dropped his guard and instantly the boy used his move to pin him. The boy won the match and became the new tournament champion. On the way home, he asked, "Sensei, how did I win the tournament with only one move?" "You won for two reasons," he answered. "First, you've almost mastered one of the most difficult throws in all of judo. And second, the only known defense for that move is for your opponent to grab your left arm."

—AUTHOR UNKNOWN

We all need that one good move in our lives, to become masterful at something difficult. What's yours? Mine is my morning jog. I didn't like it at the beginning. It took more time

and effort than I wanted to spend. But over time, little by little, it became familiar and enjoyable. Today, my day would be incomplete without it. It unfailingly clears my mind, wakes up my body, gets the blood flowing and produces endorphins to keep my stress level down. It also gives me confidence that I have an ongoing defense against heart disease. Unlike the boy in the story, it may not be an "untouchable" defense, but I know that my jog helps to strengthen my heart and ward off disease. I'm doing the right thing for my health, and that gives me a feeling of confidence and success that lasts through the day.

DAY
256

"Motivation is like nutrition. It must be taken daily and in healthy doses to keep it going."

—Norman Vincent Peale, preacher and author of *The Power of Positive Thinking*

When I eat healthy foods, I'm feeding my body well. And when I use stories, anecdotes and quotes to motivate me toward good health, I feed my mind. I need to feed both, every day.

257

Never think about quitting—unless you're talking about smoking, overeating or other toxic habits! When it comes to your health, your breaking point is often the moment of breakthrough. Many marathon runners "hit the wall" at about mile 22; they feel drained of energy and ready to give up. But seasoned runners know that if they push through the pain they'll get their second wind and experience a "runner's high" that will carry them the full 26-plus miles.

Every breaking point is a test—a test you must will yourself to pass. Don't quit. Persevere. Aim for success.

258

"Our mental and emotional diets determine our overall
energy levels, health and well-being more than we realize.
Every thought and feeling, no matter how big or small,
impacts our inner energy reserves."

—DOC CHILDRE, AUTHOR OF *TRANSFORMING STRESS*

**Doc Childre, creator of the HeartMath System (a Fortune
500 favorite), is a noted authority on optimizing human
performance and personal effectiveness by managing stess.
Reducing stress improves health, emotional well-being
and intelligence—you know that! So go ahead, take a deep
breath, relax.**

Small things count. Ask Bohn Fawkes, a B-17 pilot in World War II. During one battle he encountered flak from Nazi antiaircraft guns, but even though the gas tanks were hit, the plane did not explode. Fawkes landed it safely. The next day he asked his crew chief for the German shell; he wanted to keep it as a souvenir of his good fortune. The chief explained that a total of 11 shells had been found in the fuel tank, and none of them had exploded. Technicians opened the shells and found them clean, harmless and, with one exception, empty. The exception contained a carefully rolled piece of paper. On it a message had been scrawled in Czech: "This is all we can do for you now." A brave assembly line worker had been disarming shells when he scribbled that note. He couldn't end the war, but he could save one plane.

—Author unknown

What a moving story. The worker realized he could do something about the Nazis. And he did it! It's the same with healthy living. You may not be able to make every rule and suggestion for healthy living part of your life (at least at the beginning of your personal transformation), but you can pick two or three and make them real. Your small actions can make a big difference.

260

"If you want a guarantee, buy a toaster."

—AUTHOR UNKNOWN

I wish I could tell you that heart health is guaranteed by doing all the recommended things—eating right, exercising regularly, managing stress, not smoking, having a positive attitude. It is not. Sometimes you can do everything right and still have a bad outcome. But the chances are so much better for a good outcome when you're faithful to healthy living habits. That's why I do what I do, day in and day out. I'm playing the odds. And for over 30 years, it has worked.

DAY
261

Monitor yourself for Metabolic Syndrome, a combination of risk factors that damages coronary arteries, contributes to the buildup of plaque, promotes blood clots and triggers coronary disease. The risk profile for Metabolic Syndrome includes:

- HDL below 40 mg/dl for men or 50 mg/dl for women

- Triglyceride level above 150 mg/dl

- A potbelly: waist size 35 inches or above for women, 40 inches and above for men

- Blood pressure consistently 130/85 mm Hg or higher

- Fasting glucose of 100 mg/dl or higher, or diabetes

If you fit two of the five features above, you probably have Metabolic Syndrome. Three or more, you definitely have it. Time to talk to your doctor.

DAY
262

The humdrum can wear you down. A job that once excited you becomes monotonous; health problems rein you in; a relationship that was fresh grows stale. Some of that is inevitable. But consciously deciding to stop focusing on what's wrong will make life a whole lot sweeter.

Gonzo journalist Hunter S. Thompson reportedly observed that "Life is not a journey to the grave with the intention of arriving safely in one pretty and well-preserved piece, but to skid across the line broadside, thoroughly used up, shouting GERONIMO!"

DAY
263

"Life's ups and downs provide windows of opportunity to determine [your] values and goals. . . . Think of using all obstacles as stepping stones to build the life you want."

—Marsha Sinetar, author of *To Build the Life You Want, Create the Work You Love*

It's been said that we grow more from adversity than from ease. For me, that's been entirely true. Having heart disease at an early age was crushing, but without it I never would have written books, hosted television programs or given so many lectures—all of which have enriched my life in immeasurable ways. I'm sure I wouldn't be as healthy as I am today, either. You could say that having heart disease turned out to be one of the best things in my life!

DAY
264

Stress, stress—we never stop hearing about stress!
No surprise, what with 60-hour workweeks and long
commutes, late-night e-mails and an uncertain economy.
And stress *is* something to worry about. To begin with, it's
really bad for your heart. Stress can sabotage your good
efforts to eat well and exercise effectively, but there are
direct connections to your heart as well. Chronic stress can
raise your cholesterol, increase blood pressure, increase
blood clotting, promote Metabolic Syndrome and trigger
heart attacks. Make no mistake . . . chronic stress is a killer!

**Stress simply can't be avoided. But we can stop ourselves
from getting unduly stressed about the stresses we face!
You can take small, sensible steps to manage stress—avoid
the computer before bed, shut off the phone, take a daily
walk. One of the most effective methods for easing stress is
meditation. It involves getting in a comfortable position and
repeating a single word in your mind for a concentrated but
brief period of time. Designed to clear the mind and anchor
it in the present, meditation produces an immediate calming
effect on the nervous system. New studies at the University
of Wisconsin also show that meditation can help reduce
blood pressure and may even boost brain power.**

265

"Grow old along with me!
The best is yet to be."

—ROBERT BROWNING, POET

I could not have survived for the past three decades with heart disease if it had not been for Bernie. She is the true hero in this saga. The Browning couplet above was our hopeful mantra as over the years she prepared healthy meals, exercised with me, shared our stresses and kept me on track. As the big events in life have come along—our children's graduations, their marriages, the births of our four grandchildren, our 60th birthdays (and even applying for Medicare!), we marvel at the lifetime of answered prayers we have shared. And it's not over yet. The best is yet to come.

In the television series *The West Wing,* President Josiah Bartlett regularly ended staff meetings with two words: "What's next?" It was his way of signaling that he was finished with the issue at hand and ready to move on. The pressures and responsibilities of life in the White House demanded that he not focus on what was in the rearview mirror.

Too many of us worry about the mistakes and problems of our past, the conversations that might have happened, the road we might have walked. If that describes you, stop—that's it, simply stop. Today is all any of us can really manage.

DAY
267

"Not truth, but faith, is what keeps the world alive."

—EDNA ST. VINCENT MILLAY, POET

DAY
268

Make a truce with fast food. No question, it's contributed greatly to our epidemics of obesity, heart disease and type 2 diabetes. But from time to time we all find ourselves under the Golden Arches, and that's when we need to know how to order sensibly. In the mood for a burger, fries and something to drink? A McDonald's Quarter Pounder with Cheese, large French fries, and a 16-ounce strawberry shake will set you back 1,570 calories and 64 grams of fat. Amazing! But order a regular hamburger, small fries and 1% milk instead, and you'll be eating just 580 calories and 22.5 grams of fat.

DAY
269

David, a second-grader, was bumped while getting on the school bus and suffered a two-inch cut on his cheek. At recess he collided with another boy and lost two teeth. At noon, while sliding on ice, he fell and broke his wrist. Later, at the hospital, his father noticed that David was clutching a quarter in his good hand. David said, "I found it on the ground when I fell. This is the first quarter I ever found. This sure is my lucky day."

—MICHAEL HODGIN, AUTHOR OF *1,001 HUMOROUS ILLUSTRATIONS FOR PUBLIC SPEAKING*

Okay, maybe none of us can quite muster David's attitude, but we should all try to emulate his belief that even the worst day has something great to offer. That is the positive attitude that helps us sweep away the problems in life so that we can better focus on the essential fact: *We are here*. Don't forget to look for your lucky quarter.

DAY 270

"Every day, do something that will inch you closer to a better tomorrow."

—DOUG FIREBAUGH, MOTIVATIONAL SPEAKER

It is said that baseball is a game of inches, and it is. Just a few inches one way or another can separate a foul ball from a home run. It's the same with building a healthy lifestyle. It takes time to develop healthy eating habits like consistently ordering salmon instead of prime rib in a restaurant. Success in establishing healthy habits is the product of small steps today—inches, if you will—that add up to big strides tomorrow. So if you're just getting started and see the road to good heart health as a long one, don't be discouraged. The inches you cover today and every day may seem small, but taken together, they're a powerful push forward.

DAY
271

Take a break, for goodness sake! Some of us find this very hard to do without feeling guilty and selfish or, worse, feeling like a failure because everything on our "to do" list did not get done. Here's a news flash: *Taking a break is important for your health.* And here's another: *There will always be more to do, anyway.* So learn to delegate, to take small steps and to celebrate the small accomplishments that make up your life. Learn to take time for the people who matter; otherwise, you will lose them. Busyness destroys relationships, and no success can compensate for that.

DAY
272

Why do some people accomplish their health goals while others of equal education and capabilities do not? Often it comes down to basic principles:

1. Decide on your goal, write it down and establish a deadline. Seeing it on paper gives it permanency. Here's an example: "My exercise goal is that in 30 days I'll be walking three miles in 45 minutes, four days a week."
2. List what you need to do (buy walking shoes, for example), decide on where you will walk and line up a walking partner.
3. Convert your list into a plan and get to work on it right away. Do what you need to do today and start walking tomorrow.

It is my belief that you should do something every day to move you toward heart health. To that end, I have two sets of goals. The first contains my immediate goals: exercising daily, making smart food choices, taking time to manage stress, and so forth. But my overall goal is to maximize my heart health so that the years with my family will be long and healthy. That is a goal worth devoting my life to.

DAY
273

I am only one,
But still I am one.
I cannot do everything,
But still I can do something;
And because I cannot do everything
I will not refuse to do the something that I can do.

—EDWARD EVERETT HALE, AUTHOR AND CLERGYMAN

When I first started out on the road to a healthy lifestyle, there wasn't a lot of information on diet, exercise and stress. But applying what was there was still overwhelming. How could I do it all? It seemed so impossible to me that I didn't do anything. I was immobilized. Then I read the above poem and realized what a tragedy it would be if I did nothing just because I could do only a little. I haven't done "nothing" since!

DAY
274

Major James Nesmeth was just your average weekend golfer, shooting in the mid-to-low nineties. Then, for seven years, he completely quit the game. Never touched a club. Never set foot on a fairway. You see, Major Nesmeth spent those seven years as a prisoner of war in North Vietnam, kept in a cage 4.5 feet high and 5 feet long. But every day, to occupy his mind, he visualized playing golf at his favorite course. He experienced everything to the last detail—the fragrance of the freshly trimmed grass, the changes in weather, the grip of the club in his hands. He instructed himself as he practiced smoothing out his downswing and follow-through. Then he watched the ball arc down the exact center of the fairway, bounce a couple of times and roll to the exact spot he had selected, all in his mind. He was in no hurry. He had no place to go. So in his mind he took every step on his way to the ball, just as if he were physically on the course. It took him just as long to play 18 holes in his imagination as it would have taken in reality. Not a detail was omitted. Not once did he ever miss a shot, never a hook or a slice, never a missed putt.

—AUTHOR UNKNOWN

What did this visualization do for Major Nesmeth? After his release, he made his way to the golf course to play his first round in seven years. He shot a 74! What he had visualized in his mind, his body became capable of doing.

DAY
275

Here are the two facts that inspire me to stick with healthy exercise and eating habits:

- For every hour that you spend exercising, you can increase your life span by two hours.

- Reducing your LDL cholesterol by about 40 points—whatever number you start with—cuts your risk of heart attack by 20%.

What great information! Through exercise and diet, you can actually extend the number of healthy years you will have. Live well, live long.

The Murder of Harry D.

On the morning of his 40th birthday, Harry D. woke with a start. It was 4:00 A.M., and he was sitting on the side of his bed trembling with fear. A voice had come in a dream, whispering, "Someone is trying to kill you, Harry."

With shaky hands, Harry lit up his first cigarette of the day and pondered the situation. His wife was now awake also, so he shared the horrifying message with her. "It's too terrible to think about," she said. "Let's have breakfast instead." But Harry couldn't shake his concern as he salted his fried eggs and carefully mopped up the bacon drippings with his buttered toast. *Who would want to kill me?* he thought as he stirred sugar and cream into his coffee and lit another smoke.

He continued to ponder the question on the drive to the office. But weaving through lanes, beating stoplights and shouting at other drivers was too frustrating to maintain concentration. Nor could he find time at work. Meetings, decisions, deadlines, phone calls . . . everything always piled up. It wasn't until he was rapidly inhaling his cheeseburger and fries at lunch that the terror of his position became clear to him. It was all he could do to finish his chocolate shake.

He worked until 7:00 P.M. as usual. Drove home fast as usual. Had his two cocktails as usual. Ate a hearty meal as usual. Studied business reports as usual. And took his usual two sleeping pills to get his usual six hours of sleep. As time went on, Harry began to take comfort in this routine. Apparently, he was outfoxing the would-be murderer. "Whoever is trying to kill me," he said proudly to his wife, "hasn't gotten me yet. I'm too smart for him." "Yes, you are, Harry," she replied while slicing his second helping of prime rib.

The months turned into years and Harry continued on, certain that he was outsmarting his murderer. But, as it must to all men, death came at last. Harry D. was 51 years old. It came at dinner while he was watching *Monday Night Football,* the closest he ever got to exercise. He simply fell over into his fettuccine Alfredo. His grief-stricken wife demanded a full autopsy. It showed coronary artery blockages, elevated cholesterol and triglycerides, emphysema, ulcers, cirrhosis of the liver, hardening of the arteries, pulmonary edema, obesity and a touch of lung cancer. "How glad he would have been to know," said his widow, smiling through her tears, "that he died of natural causes."

Sadly, we all know too many Harrys. That's why I wrote this story. Maybe it will make you listen up—even if your name is Tom or Dick.

DAY

277

"Whether you think that you can or you think that you can't, you are usually right."

—HENRY FORD, AUTOMOBILE MANUFACTURER

DAY

278

Here's an idea for anyone who's just starting a weight-training program: Why not try both weight machines *and* free weights? Machines allow for slow, concentrated movements, and you won't need anyone to "spot" you when you lift. Free weights (dumbbells and barbells), which force you to control an object while you lift it, more closely mimic everyday activities. (But be careful to have someone monitor you when you're lifting a barbell, particularly at the beginning.) Whichever you do, remember to take at least 48 hours off to rest your muscles after a session.

279

"The question is not whether we will die,
but how we will live."

—JOAN BORYSENKO, PSYCHOLOGIST AND AUTHOR OF *MINDING THE BODY,
   MENDING THE MIND*

Everybody lives, everybody dies. What counts is what we do
with the time in between. So whatever you do, do it to the
best of your ability. Make today's session on the elliptical
trainer the best ever! Serve your grilled chicken elegantly, on
the good china. Live with style, grace and purpose.

280

There are two days in every week that we shouldn't worry about—two days that should be kept free from fear and apprehension. One is yesterday, with its mistakes and cares, its faults and blunders, its aches and pains. But yesterday has gone, passed forever beyond our control. All the money in the world cannot bring it back, and we cannot undo a single act we performed or erase a single word we've said. The other day we shouldn't worry about is tomorrow; that, too, is beyond our control. Tomorrow's sun will rise either in splendor or masked by clouds, but it will rise. And until it does, we have no stake in tomorrow, since it is yet unborn. This leaves just one day—today.

—AUTHOR UNKNOWN

We can most effectively fight the battles of just one day. It's only when we add the burdens of yesterday and the worries of tomorrow that we break down. Yesterday is done and gone, but you may be able to do something today to help with tomorrow. If you're stressing about tomorrow, take time to discern if you can do anything today to help alleviate that stress. If you are to give a speech tomorrow, working on your remarks today will help to ease your concern. But if you're worried because no one may come to your talk, that's something beyond your control. Let it go.

DAY
281

"The state of your life is nothing more than a reflection of your state of mind."

—WAYNE DYER, PH.D., AUTHOR OF *YOUR ERRONEOUS ZONES*

DAY
282

"I woke up early today, excited over all I get to do before the clock strikes midnight. I have responsibilities to fulfill. My job is to choose what kind of day I am going to have. I can complain because the weather is rainy or I can be thankful that the grass is getting watered for free. I can grumble about my health or I can rejoice that I am alive. I can cry because roses have thorns or I can celebrate that thorns have roses. I can whine because I have to go to work or I can shout for joy because I have a job to do."

—AUTHOR UNKNOWN

Each today is new, stretching ahead of me, waiting to be shaped. And here I am, the sculptor who gets to do the shaping. What will the day be like? It's all up to me. What kind of day is yours shaping up to be?

DAY

283

Portion size—that's the nasty little secret behind weight gain. With plates becoming so big (from an average of 9.5 inches in the 1970s to 14.5 inches today) and with most restaurant meals supersized, the servings are usually much too large. And if you eat more than the proper portion— even of healthy food—you'll put on weight. Here are some visualizations that may make it easier for you to keep your portions under control:

- 3 ounces of meat, poultry or fish = a bar of soap, a checkbook or a deck of playing cards

- 2 tablespoons of peanut butter = a golf ball

- 1 medium bagel = a hockey puck

- 3 ounces of hamburger = the lid of a medium-size jar of mayonnaise

- ½ cup of cooked vegetables, cut fruit, cooked rice or pasta = a cupcake liner

- 1 cup of raw, leafy vegetables or dry cereal = a baseball

- 1 ounce of cheese = 4 dice

284

"Each morning when I open my eyes, I say to myself: I, not events, have the power to make me happy or unhappy today. I can choose which it shall be. Yesterday is dead; tomorrow hasn't yet arrived. I have just one day, today, and I'm going to be happy in it."

—GROUCHO MARX, COMEDIAN

It's so interesting to me to hear or read really smart and insightful ideas from comedians. These thoughts pack a double punch. First you get to remember the comics' funnier moments. I'm a big fan of Groucho's gag: "I'm not feeling very well. I need a doctor immediately. Ring the nearest golf course!" Then you get to contemplate the intelligence that makes true humor possible.

DAY
285

And speaking of funny, laughter is among the best medicines for protecting your heart. Truly. A wide body of research suggests that laughter can be a powerful antidote to stress by relaxing the body and triggering the release of endorphins. But two new studies show that laughter can be powerful medicine by improving blood flow, which can help to ward off high blood pressure.

Laughter promotes deep breathing, which makes your body relax, and that in turn relieves stress. You can get the same deep breathing results from yoga, tai chi and, of course, deep breathing exercises. Says Dr. Paul McGhee, an expert on laughter as medicine, "Your sense of humor is one of the most powerful tools you have to make certain that your daily mood and emotional state support good health."

DAY
286

"If you don't like something, change it. If you can't change it, change your attitude. Don't complain."

—MAYA ANGELOU, AUTHOR AND POET

DAY
287

Almost every minute that you're awake, you have a conversation with yourself. Some are brief; some are detailed and lengthy. And those internal dialogues are the most important communications you have. They affect your success in life more than any other factor. In these silent conversations, you solve problems—or create them. You judge, praise or disparage yourself. You dwell on past mistakes or you plan future achievements.

In the computer world, *GIGO* means "garbage in, garbage out." Your mind works the same way. Obviously, the more positive and forward-looking your talk, the stronger and better prepared you become.

288

Imagine a magic potion that could make you feel great and cut your risk of getting heart disease, cancer or diabetes in half. People would be willing to spend hundreds, even thousands of dollars for it. But it's already available . . . and free. I know you know what it is—regular physical activity. So go get some!

289

"It's always too early to quit."

—NORMAN VINCENT PEALE, PREACHER AND AUTHOR OF *THE POWER OF POSITIVE THINKING*

I met Florence Chadwick, the first woman to swim the English Channel, on a television show in San Diego. She talked about having clear goals and used her attempt to swim from Catalina Island to the California coast as an example. The fog was so thick that she couldn't see anything in front of her. Her mother and trainer offered encouragement from one of the boats and they told her it wasn't much farther. But all she could see was fog. With only a half-mile to go, for the first time in her life she quit. It wasn't fatigue or the cold water that defeated her; it was that fog. She was unable to see her goal. Two months later, she tried again. This time, despite the same dense fog, she swam with her goal clearly pictured in her mind and made it, becoming the first woman to swim the Catalina Channel. "The message," she said, "is to have a clear goal in your mind and never to quit."

DAY 290

Reading the nutrition facts on processed and packaged foods is a lot easier than it was a while ago, when labels contained more advertising than information. Now you can just look in the upper left-hand corner and find the number of servings, calories per serving, fat, saturated fat, trans fat, sodium, fiber and sugars. But don't forget to read the list of ingredients so you can determine what has been added. The fewer ingredients, the better the food is for your health. The best way to eat, of course, is to avoid processed foods in favor of whole foods—particularly fruits, whole grains, vegetables and fish.

DAY
291

"A goal is a dream with a deadline."

—NAPOLEON HILL, AUTHOR OF *THINK AND GROW RICH*

Remember where this book started—with that important distinction between a "can do" and a "will do" attitude? When I was a "can do" person, I had fitness plans and goals but rarely got around to getting started. When I became a "will do" person, my goals took on an urgency. Only then was I able to get moving.

DAY
292

Be wary of dietary supplements, particularly those claiming to burn fat, build muscle or boost metabolism. They're a multibillion-dollar industry, but these supplements are not regulated by the Food and Drug Administration for safety or effectiveness. The FDA steps in only after receiving reports of illness. So be skeptical. If a claim is too good to be true, don't listen. A few supplements are vetted, such as fish oil pills for those with heart disease, vitamin D and calcium for many people, and folic acid for women of childbearing age. But contrary to the claims that they can ward off aging, guaranteeing weight loss and curing Alzheimer's, most dietary supplements are ineffective and some are harmful.

DAY
293

A chicken and a pig were walking down the street and saw a sign in a restaurant window: HAM AND EGGS, $2.00. "Look at that," said the chicken proudly. "I'm involved." The pig studied the sign for a long time and said, "For you, it's involvement. For me, it's total commitment."

I thought hard about not using this cute story because I didn't want to equate "total commitment" with the pig's demise. But, come on! Having health and fitness as lifetime goals is much more than involvement. It *is* total commitment . . . but in a good way!

294

"People think I'm disciplined. It is not discipline. It is devotion. There is a great difference."

—LUCIANO PAVAROTTI, OPERA SINGER

I can identify so much with this quote. When I began to change my diet to healthier eating, it took great discipline to pass up cheeseburgers, ice cream and French fries for poultry, fish and vegetables. I longed for my old way of eating, but discipline kept me on course. On the six-month anniversary of eating very healthy, I decided to "celebrate" by ordering a rib-eye steak in a restaurant. I could hardly wait to eat it. Finally, it was served and the heady aroma made my mouth water. But what a disappointment! The fat from the meat coated my mouth and tongue. It felt like a layer of Vaseline. I couldn't wait to get back to healthier foods. Over time, that discipline changed into a devotion. Today I eat healthy foods (in our cookbooks, Bernie and I offer more than a thousand recipes) because I want to, not because I am especially disciplined.

DAY
295

I read a story about a man who took his two small children to the circus. As they wandered around, looking at the circus animals, they came upon the elephants. These huge creatures had no cages like the lions and tigers. No chains. They were held only by small ropes tied to their front legs. Obviously the elephants could, at any time, break away from their bonds, but they did not. The man asked a trainer why these magnificent animals just stood there, making no attempt to escape. "When they're very young and much smaller," he said, "this size rope is enough to hold them. As they grow up, they're conditioned to believe they cannot break away. They think the rope can still hold them, so they never try to break free."

—AUTHOR UNKNOWN

If you don't think you can break your bonds, you will be stuck where you are—forever.

DAY

296

Although Henri Matisse was nearly 28 years younger than Auguste Renoir, the two great artists were dear friends and frequent companions. When Renoir was confined to his home during the last decade of his life, Matisse visited him daily. Renoir, almost paralyzed by arthritis, continued to paint despite his infirmities. One day, as Matisse watched his friend working in his studio, fighting torturous pain with each brushstroke, he blurted out, "Auguste, why do you continue to paint when you're in such agony?" Renoir answered simply: "The beauty remains; the pain passes." And so, almost to his dying day, Renoir put paint to canvas.

—AUTHOR UNKNOWN

Persistence overcoming pain, producing beauty: a message for art . . . and for life.

DAY
297

"For a long time it had seemed to me that life was about to begin—real life. But there was always some obstacle in the way, something to be got through first, some unfinished business, time still to be served, a debt to be paid. Then life would begin. At last it dawned on me that these obstacles were my life."

—FR. ALFRED D'SOUZA, WRITER

DAY
298

"Don't wait until everything is just right. It will never be perfect. There will always be challenges, obstacles and less than perfect conditions. So what. Get started now. With each step you take, you will grow stronger and stronger, more and more skilled, more and more self-confident and more and more successful."

—MARK VICTOR HANSEN, COAUTHOR OF *CHICKEN SOUP FOR THE SOUL*

DAY
299

A young student approached the famous French scientist and philosopher Blaise Pascal and declared, "If I had your brains, I would be a better person." Pondering the depth of this statement, Pascal paused momentarily before replying, "Be a better person and you will have my brains."

—AUTHOR UNKNOWN

How often have I heard someone say, "If I were in better shape, I'd be at the gym every day"? But the opposite is true. Go to the gym every day and you will be in great shape.

DAY
300

"You can't cross the sea merely by standing and staring at the water."

—RABINDRANATH TAGORE, POET

We live near the water in Washington State, and let me tell you, that water can be mighty cold! I love watching my grandkids run down the sand in their bare feet, letting the water just touch their toes before they scoot back to the safety of their parents' arms. Then it's back to the water, where the kids let the tide lap up just a little higher on their legs. And as they stand there laughing, thrilled with their own bravery, I practically weep for the glory of the possibility we all hold within us.

Picture this: You're in a restaurant, looking at the dessert menu, and everything sounds so tempting. But then think about it—is it the actual food that's enticing you, or the descriptions you're reading? If, like most people, you're more likely to order Dark Chocolate Torte or a French Vanilla Cheesecake with Strawberry Glaze than regular chocolate cake or cheesecake, take a minute to decide if you're being bamboozled into wanting something you could just as easily do without.

Of course we should indulge ourselves sometimes, even on a healthy diet. I love to have a restaurant dessert now and then—but I never order a whole one just for me. Bernie and I split one serving; we still get the treat but we don't end up stuffed . . . or feeling guilty.

DAY
302

"When I look back on all these worries, I remember the story of the old man who said on his deathbed that he had had a lot of trouble in his life, most of which had never happened."

—Winston Churchill, prime minister of Great Britain

If you worry about the recipe not working, you'll never cook the delicious dish. If you worry about pulling a muscle, you'll never take a walk. If you worry about always being out of time, you'll never have any for yourself.

Go ahead—just do it, whatever "it" is!

DAY
303

There's a bank that credits your account each morning with $86,400, carries over no balance from day to day, allows you to keep no cash balance and every evening cancels whatever part of the amount you had failed to use during the day. How are you going to use it? Draw out every cent, of course! We all have a bank just like this, and its name is TIME. Every morning, it credits you with 86,400 seconds. Every night it writes off as lost whatever you have failed to invest to good purpose. It carries over no balance, allows no overdraft. Each day, it opens a new account for you; each night, it burns the records of the day. There is no going back, no drawing against tomorrow. You must live in the present on today's deposits.

—AUTHOR UNKNOWN

The clock is running. Make the most of today. And invest wisely for the maximum return in health, happiness and success.

DAY
304

If your doctor tells you that you're at risk for diabetes, eat more fruit and leafy green vegetables and go easy on fruit juice. A team from the Tulane School of Public Health and Tropical Medicine and the Harvard School of Public Health analyzed 18 years' worth of diet and health data from 71,346 nurses who participated in the Nurses' Health Study from 1984 to 2002. They found that eating just one serving of green leafy vegetables or three servings of fruit a day reduces the risk of developing type 2 diabetes, while drinking one serving of fruit juice a day increased the risk. Bottom line: People with risk factors for diabetes should fill up on leafy greens like lettuce, kale and spinach and whole fruits like apples, bananas, oranges and watermelon rather than drink fruit juices, which deliver a big sugar load in a liquid form that gets absorbed rapidly. In addition to emphasizing the importance of eating whole fruits and green leafy vegetables to prevent diabetes, researchers recommend replacing refined grains and white potatoes with whole fruit or green leafy vegetable servings. White flours and potatoes have been associated with an increased risk of diabetes.

305

Motivational speaker Charles Plumb was once a navy pilot in Vietnam. After 75 combat missions, his plane was shot down. Plumb ejected, parachuted into enemy hands and spent six years as a POW. A few years later, he tells his audience, he was walking through a hotel lobby with his wife when a man stopped him and said, "You're Plumb! You flew jet fighters in Vietnam from the *Kitty Hawk*. You were shot down!" "How in the world did you know that?" asked Plumb. "I packed your parachute," the man replied. "I guess it worked!" Plumb exclaimed, "It sure did. If your chute hadn't worked, I wouldn't be here today!" Plumb says he couldn't sleep that night. He kept thinking about that man. "I kept wondering what he might have looked like back then in a navy uniform. I wonder how many times I might have seen him and not even said 'Good morning, how are you' or anything like that because, you see, I was a fighter pilot and he was just a sailor." Plumb then began to think of the many hours that ordinary sailor had spent weaving and folding the silk of each chute, holding in his hands each time the fate of an unknown person. At that point in his program, Plumb usually asks his audience, "Who's packing your parachute?"

Recognize your many supporters on the road to fitness— your spouse, family, friends and medical team. Don't forget to thank your wife for cooking a healthy dinner, or the trainer

at the gym who showed you a new exercise, or the nurse who got you in to see the doctor when his schedule was full. As you go through this week, this month, this year, appreciate the people who pack your parachute.

DAY
306

"Pain is temporary. It may last a minute or an hour, or a day or a year. But eventually it will subside and something else will take its place. If I quit, however, it lasts forever."

—LANCE ARMSTRONG, CHAMPION CYCLIST

Even in the face of cancer, Lance Armstrong didn't quit. That's the mark of a true champion. Not many of us will wear the yellow jersey on the Tour de France, but we are champions every day that we practice healthy habits.

307

"If you could kick the person in the pants responsible for most of your trouble, you wouldn't sit for a month."

—THEODORE ROOSEVELT, 26TH PRESIDENT OF THE UNITED STATES

It's all too easy to blame other people or circumstances for everything that gets in the way of maintaining healthy habits: "My schedule kept me from the gym," or "I'm traveling and forgot to pack my running shoes," or "Why did you make such a delicious dinner? I *had* to have seconds." No outside forces keep us from doing what we need to do. We're the ones to blame. Next time you mess up, look in the mirror, accept responsibility for any setback (and of course there will be setbacks!) and recommit to a healthier lifestyle.

DAY
308

Thirty minutes a day. Just 30 minutes of physical activity daily will help to keep you healthy. That includes gardening and yard work, which can give you a cardiovascular workout and strengthen your bones and muscles. Digging, laying sod, raking and using a push mower can burn more energy than brisk walking. You just have to know how to get more out of gardening:

- Space out your yard work over several days rather than doing it in bruising seasonal marathons.

- Allow at least 30 minutes for each yard work session.

- Use an old-fashioned manual mower. It will help you burn lots of calories (and it's better for the environment than a power mower).

- Use a rake, not a power leaf blower, for a good upper-body workout.

An American investment banker and a Mexican fisherman were returning from a two-hour fishing trip. The American asked, "But what do you do with the rest of your time?"

The fisherman answered, "Well, I sleep late, fish a little, play with my children, take a siesta with my wife, and stroll into the village in the evening to sip wine and play guitar with my *amigos*."

The American said, "I am a Harvard MBA, and I could help you. You should spend more time fishing. With the proceeds, you could buy a bigger boat. With the proceeds from the bigger boat, you could buy several boats. Eventually you would have a fleet of fishing boats. Instead of selling your catch to a middleman, you would sell directly to the processor; eventually you would open your own cannery and control the product, processing and distribution. You would leave this small coastal village and move to Mexico City, then Los Angeles and then New York, where you would preside over your thriving enterprise. It would take 15 to 20 years."

"But what then?" asked the fisherman.

The businessman laughed and said, "That's the best part. When the time was right, you would announce an IPO and sell your company stock to the public and become very rich. You would make millions! Then you would retire. You would move to a small coastal fishing village where you would sleep late, fish a little, play with your kids, take a siesta with your wife, and stroll into the village in the evening to sip wine and play your guitar with your *amigos*."

—AUTHOR UNKNOWN

Know how you want your journey to end before you start walking. Sometimes you'll discover that you might as well stay home.

DAY
310

"Even ordinary effort over time yields extraordinary results."

—AUTHOR UNKNOWN

These words perfectly sum up my efforts to live healthy. I've never gone to extremes. I've never eaten a no-fat diet or run a marathon, lifted huge amounts of weight at the gym or gone to Tibet to meditate. I've always taken a moderate approach and made what you might call an ordinary effort. But that ordinary effort has allowed me to manage my heart disease for over 30 years. And that is an extraordinary result.

DAY
311

"If you love life, don't waste time,
for time is what life is made up of."

—BRUCE LEE, MARTIAL ARTIST

DAY
312

There was an important job to be done and Everybody was sure Somebody would do it. Anybody could have done it, but Nobody did. Somebody got angry about that because it was Everybody's job. Everybody thought Anybody could do it, but Nobody realized that Everybody would not do it. It ended up that Everybody blamed Somebody when Nobody did what Anybody could have done.

—AUTHOR UNKNOWN

The responsibility for how you live your life starts and stops with you. Don't wait for Somebody to step in on your behalf.

DAY
313

It's not just overweight that causes health problems; there's also the matter of where your body stores that extra fat. The link between overweight and heart disease is particularly strong if excess fat is carried around the middle. People with wide hips and flat bellies (a "pear shape") may be overweight, but the extra weight does not seem to increase their cardiac risk as much as that of people with narrow hips and potbellies (an "apple shape"). Perhaps because abdominal fat is more metabolically active than fat stored in thighs, hips and buttocks, "apples" are three to five times more likely than "pears" to suffer heart attacks. "Apples" are also much more likely to have high cholesterol, hypertension and diabetes. You can determine if you're at risk by measuring your waist just above the navel. The American Heart Association defines a high-risk waistline as 35 inches or more for women and 40 inches or more for men. What can you do about it if you're an apple? Reduce that excess body fat by eating fewer calories (less fat and sugar, more veggies, smaller portions) and by exercising daily (many experts call for brisk walking one hour a day).

DAY
314

Track your daily mileage with a pedometer, one of the greatest motivators ever to clip on a belt! To meet the recommended goal of at least 30 minutes of physical activity every day, aim for a total of 10,000 steps. At the beginning, you may find that you have to walk the dog around the block a few more times to get there, but pretty soon it will be second nature.

Inactive people take between 2,000 and 4,000 steps per day; moderately active people, between 5,000 and 7,000 steps per day; active people, at least 10,000 (roughly five miles). Those 10,000 steps burn off about 500 calories—just in case you want a little motivation.

DAY
315

Try an experiment: Turn off the TV news. It often presents the day's headlines in a lurid and sensationalized way so that instead of bringing clarity, it increases our stress and anxiety. Every day we are subjected to unforgettable images of violence and destruction—school shootings, war, floods, financial disasters. But if you rely on written reporting, you're more likely to get a calmer, balanced account.

DAY
316

Make good health your absolute number one priority. The single most important thing I've learned in the three decades since bypass surgery is this: If you don't take time for health today, you'll have to make time for illness tomorrow.

Shay, a physically handicapped 10-year-old boy, and his father walked past a park where some boys were playing baseball. Shay asked, "Do you think they would let me play?" Shay's father thought the boys probably wouldn't like the idea, but he felt that playing with them would give his son a much-needed sense of belonging, so he went ahead and asked. "We're losing by six runs and the game is in the eighth inning," said one of the boys. "He can be on our team and we'll try to put him in to bat in the ninth." Shay struggled over to the team's bench and, with a broad smile, put on a team shirt. At the bottom of the eighth inning, his team had scored but was still behind by three. At the top of the ninth, Shay put on a glove and played right field. Even though no hits came his way, he was overjoyed just to be in the game. In the bottom of the ninth, Shay's team scored again. Now, with two outs and the bases loaded, Shay was scheduled to come up next. Would they let him bat and maybe give away their chance to win the game? They did, even though they were aware that Shay didn't even know how to hold the bat properly, much less connect with the ball.

Shay stepped up to the plate, and the pitcher realized that the other team had chosen to put aside the idea of winning for the sake of Shay. He moved in a few steps to lob the ball softly enough for Shay to at least make contact. Shay swung clumsily and missed. The pitcher again took a few steps forward and tossed the ball softly. Shay swung at the pitch and hit a slow grounder right back to the pitcher. The pitcher picked it up and could easily have thrown to first and gotten the last out, but instead he threw the ball right over the first baseman's head. Everyone from the stands and both teams started yelling, "Shay, run to first! Run to first!"

Never in his life had Shay run that far, but he made it to first base. Everyone yelled, "Run to second, run to second!" Catching his breath, Shay awkwardly ran toward second, struggling to make it to the base. The right fielder had the ball now and could have thrown to the second baseman for the tag, but he threw to third instead, high and far over the baseman's head. Shay rounded second behind the baserunner who represented the tying run.

Now everyone was screaming, "Shay, Shay, Shay, all the way, Shay!" The opposing shortstop ran to help him by turning him in the right direction and shouting, "Run to third, Shay, run to third!" As Shay rounded third, the boys from both teams and all the spectators were on their feet screaming, "Shay, run home! Run home!" Shay ran home, stepped on the plate and was cheered as the hero who hit the grand slam and won the game for his team.

—AUTHOR UNKNOWN

Young Shay would never forget what it felt like to be a hero that day—nor would the other boys. Be a hero to your family by doing what you need to do, today, to achieve heart health.

DAY
318

"I do not try to dance better than anyone else. I only try to dance better than myself."

—MIKHAIL BARYSHNIKOV, BALLET DANCER

Life is not a competition; neither is living healthy. It's not about who can eat the most salads or walk the most miles. It's about trying to be personally better today than you were yesterday—or at least as good!

DAY
319

"Stress can lead to obesity. When they're stressed, people often comfort themselves by eating foods that are rich in fat, sugar and calories. These foods act as an edible tranquilizer—nature's way of getting you to feel better!"

—JUDITH WURTMAN, PH.D., NUTRITION EXPERT

Just remember that exercise can make you feel better, too—and without any harmful side effects. People who exercise regularly produce endorphins, brain chemicals that make you feel happy, relaxed and in control. The next time you're feeling wound up, go for a jog and run right by the ice cream shop!

DAY
320

We are sleep-deprived workaholics. According to the National Sleep Foundation, only about a third of us sleep the recommended seven to eight hours a night and 40% say they have trouble staying awake on the job. We live in a chronically overtired society where instead of working to live, we are living to work, a practice that has a profound impact on our health. Evidence is mounting that decreased sleep is associated with heart disease, diabetes, cancer, obesity and depression. "Getting enough sleep should be considered just as important as eating a healthy diet and exercising," says Dr. Michael Sateia, medical director of the Sleep Disorders Service at Dartmouth-Hitchcock Medical Center.

Ever since I was a teenager, I just knew that lying around must be good for you. Go ahead: Get those zzz's!

321

About a thousand years ago, a wise man came upon some men working. He asked one of them, "What are you doing, my good man?" The man looked up. "I'm working," he said curtly and went back to his labors. Not satisfied with the answer, the sage approached a second workman and asked the same question. "You can see. I'm breaking stones," he replied. The sage was made of stern stuff and he wasn't leaving without an answer, so he walked over to a third workman and asked him the question. "I'm building a temple," said the workman, smiling. The incident opened the sage's eyes. While all three of the workers were breaking up stones, in their minds they were not doing the same jobs. The third workman was working for a cause much larger than himself, and it showed in his attitude and his approach to work.

—AUTHOR UNKNOWN

You can just do a day's work, or you can build your equivalent of a temple—a career, a team, an organization, a nation.

DAY
322

"When I stand before God at the end of my life, I would hope that I would not have a single bit of talent left and could say, 'I used everything you gave me.'"

—ERMA BOMBECK, COLUMNIST

I'm with Erma! I want to give it my all. I'd like God to say, "Good work! You didn't leave anything on the table."

DAY
323

"I learned that the only way you are going to get anywhere in life is to work hard at it. Whether you're a musician, a writer, an athlete or a businessman, there is no getting around it. If you do, you'll win—if you don't, you won't."

—BRUCE JENNER, OLYMPIC TRACK-AND-FIELD CHAMPION

Lessons from an Oyster

There once was an oyster
Whose story I tell,
Who found that some sand
Had got into his shell.

It was only a grain
But it gave him great pain,
For oysters have feelings
Although they're so plain.

Now, did he berate
The harsh workings of fate
That had brought him
To such a deplorable state?

Did he curse at the government,
Cry for election,
And claim that the sea should
Have given him protection?

"No," he said to himself
As he lay on a shell,
Since I cannot remove it,
I shall try to improve it.

Now the years have rolled around,
As the years always do,
And he came to his ultimate
Destiny . . . stew.

And the small grain of sand
That had bothered him so
Was a beautiful pearl
All richly aglow.

Now the tale has a moral,
For isn't it grand
What an oyster can do
With a morsel of sand?

What couldn't we do
If we'd only begin
With some of the things
That get under our skin.

—AUTHOR UNKNOWN

DAY
325

People often quit trying in the face of obstacles. But in reality, obstacles are frequently the secret ingredient in the recipe for success. That's because every obstacle you encounter can bring you one step closer to success—if you persist. Try visualizing an obstacle not as an impenetrable concrete wall, but rather as a temporary barrier. Have faith in your ability to knock it down. Tap into your desire to succeed. Before you know it . . . the wall has vanished. The next time you face an obstacle, don't give up, don't quit. Instead, stop and ponder these questions: "If I were to overcome this obstacle, what would I accomplish? Would toppling this wall help me to achieve what I want? Would it allow me to be where I want to be?"

If the answer to the last two questions is yes, figure out what it will take to break that obstacle so that you can continue on your path to success. If the answer is no, don't struggle to overcome the barrier. Just turn your back on it and walk away.

DAY
326

"The way to get started is to quit talking and begin doing."

—WALT DISNEY, ANIMATOR AND DIRECTOR

DAY
327

Put whole grains on your menu. Low in fat, rich in protein, B vitamins and vitamin E, high in fiber and low in calories, they represent a nutritional bonanza. Most of them provide 3 to 10 grams of fiber per quarter-cup, but only about 200 calories. And don't restrict yourself to whole-grain breakfast cereals. Incorporate whole grains such as brown rice, wheat, corn, barley, bulgur and whole-wheat couscous into your other meals—sustaining and delicious.

DAY
328

Long ago in a faraway village, there was a place called the House of 1,000 Mirrors. A small, happy dog learned of this place and decided to visit. On arrival, he bounced up the stairs to the doorway of the house. To his great surprise, he found himself staring at 1,000 other small, happy dogs with their tails wagging just as fast as his. He smiled a friendly smile and was answered with 1,000 smiles just as friendly. As he left the house, he thought to himself, *This is a wonderful place. I will come back and visit it often.* Meanwhile, another small dog, who was not as happy as the first one, decided to visit the house. He slowly climbed the stairs and hung his head low as he looked into the door. When he saw 1,000 unfriendly dogs staring back at him, he growled at them and was horrified to see 1,000 small dogs growling back at him. As he left, he thought to himself, *That is a horrible place. I will never go back there again.*

—AUTHOR UNKNOWN

The faces of people we encounter can serve as mirrors for us. What kinds of reflections do you see in the faces of the people you meet? Are they positive or negative?

DAY
329

"Too often we get distracted by what is outside our control. You can't do anything about yesterday. The door to the past has been shut and the key thrown away. You can do nothing about tomorrow. It is yet to come. However, tomorrow is in large part determined by what you do today. So make today a masterpiece. You have control over that."

—JOHN WOODEN, BASKETBALL COACH

I've made this point before and will do so again—it's that important. It is critical to live your life for today, with no recriminations about yesterday, no anxieties about tomorrow. Today is all that you have. But it is also essential to set the tone for how you will live today in your mind. A few minutes in the morning, spent with a moving story or a motivational quote, can help you to focus on what to do and how to do it . . . today!

DAY
330

Pay attention to the amounts you eat. Researchers at Pennsylvania State University found that men served 2.5 cups of macaroni and cheese ate 1.9 cups. But when they were served a 5-cup portion, they ate 2.5 cups. Participants said they were equally full after each meal regardless of the amount they had eaten.

Bernie says, "That's just because they're men!" I don't usually argue with Bernie, but women are just as susceptible to the dangers presented by huge portions. Don't allow yourself to fall into the trap. If you're served too large a portion, cut it to the appropriate size before you even start eating. If you're in a restaurant, ask the waiter to take it away and put it in a doggie bag for you. If you're a guest at someone's house, just push the extra portion to the side. No one will know the difference—except for you.

DAY
331

"Don't wait. The time will never be just right."

—NAPOLEON HILL, AUTHOR OF *THINK AND GROW RICH*

And what you do will probably never be perfect. But at least you'll be doing!

DAY
332

Two frogs fell into a bucket of milk. Both tried to jump to freedom, but the sides of the bucket were steep. Seeing little chance of escape, the first frog soon despaired and stopped jumping. He sank to the bottom of the bucket and drowned. The second frog also saw no chance of success, but he didn't stop trying. Even though each jump seemed to reach the same inadequate height, he kept on struggling. Eventually, his persistent efforts churned some of the milk into butter. As the surface of the milk hardened, he managed to get his footing and leap out of the bucket.

—AUTHOR UNKNOWN

If you never quit trying, you may be surprised by the unexpected good things that will come your way.

DAY
333

"How many a man has thrown up his hands at a time when a little more effort, a little more patience, would have achieved success?"

—ELBERT HUBBARD, PHILOSOPHER AND WRITER

Wally Pipp, the regular first baseman for the New York Yankees, had the flu. He was replaced by a young player named Lou Gehrig. Gehrig played so well that Pipp lost his job as a starter. A couple of years later Gehrig had the flu, but instead of staying home in bed, he came to the ballpark and played. Soon the flu passed and he kept on playing and playing . . . for 2,130 consecutive games. See what a little more effort on Lou Gehrig's part allowed him to accomplish.

DAY
334

"Our greatest glory consists not in never falling, but in rising every time we fall."

—OLIVER GOLDSMITH, AUTHOR AND POET

DAY
335

Which has more fat and calories: a tablespoon of salad
dressing or a tablespoon of hot fudge? You're wrong if you
picked the fudge. Commercial salad dressings are about
90% fat, or about 9 grams of fat per tablespoon. To put this
in perspective, a single packet of Thousand Island dressing
at McDonald's contains more fat than one cup of Ben &
Jerry's premium chocolate ice cream! A smart way to dress
a salad is with balsamic vinegar mixed with a bit of olive oil.
If you use commercial dressings, be sure to try one of the
many nonfat or "light" versions. Nonfat dressings control
fat and calories but differ greatly in taste. Experiment.
"Light" dressings will save, on average, about 7 grams of fat
per tablespoon over regular dressings. However, fat grams
and calories can add up rapidly even with "light" dressing
if you use it too freely.

If you do use regular dressing, a good tip is to serve
it on the side. Dip your fork into the dressing, then eat
the salad. You'll get all the flavor of the dressing while
minimizing your fat and calorie intake.

336

All of us, even the most adventurous eaters, return time and again to our own food, our own favorite recipes. So, if you end up preparing healthy food that isn't familiar or flavorful, you simply won't want to eat it . . . which will lead you to eating food that is not so healthy. Here's the trick: Rewrite your favorite recipes by substituting ingredients that are lower in fat and calories. There's no need worrying about learning to create a hundred new low-fat recipes; indeed, most American families prepare only 12 recipes 80% of the time. Stick with the foods that already have your family's seal of approval. Just make them healthier.

DAY
337

"Only those who do nothing at all make no mistakes . . . but that would be a mistake."

—AUTHOR UNKNOWN

Don't be afraid of trying to live a heart-healthy lifestyle because you might make a mistake. I remember running in a 10K race with thousands of other people, including a number of my friends. It was just a year or two after my bypass, and I was anxious to show everyone that I had fully recovered. I started out fast—in fact, too fast—and at the 8K mark I was out of steam. I had to walk to finish the race. All the training, all the preparation—it seemed like such a waste. I was almost ready to give up on exercise until I realized that yes, it was a mistake to start out at that pace, but that "mistake" just became part of my experience. It would be filed mentally for me to use the next time I ran this race. As musician Robert Fripp says, "There are no mistakes, save one: the failure to learn from a mistake."

DAY
338

Have some tea today. Drinking at least one cup of green or black tea daily can significantly cut your risk of heart attack and stroke. The benefit may be due to flavonoids, powerful plant chemicals that protect your blood vessel linings from injury and inflammation. Other good sources are fruits, vegetables and red wine.

DAY
339

"The best day of your life is the one on which you decide your life is your own. No apologies or excuses. No one to lean on, rely on or blame. The gift is yours—it is an amazing journey—and you alone are responsible for the quality of it. This is the day your life really begins."

—BOB MOAWAD, MOTIVATIONAL SPEAKER

My friend Bob, who died a few years ago, was a great speaker, and his wisdom continues to inspire me. Self-responsibility is the primary building block for living in good health.

DAY
340

A lady whose friend was a chronic worrier said to her one day, "Do you realize that eighty percent of the things you worry about never happen?"

"See," her friend replied, "it works!"

Have you noticed that all roads lead to the refrigerator when you're worried? Have you also realized that fretting often makes you too tired—at least mentally—to exercise? The key question to ask yourself is this: Is there anything I can do to alleviate my worry? If you're late for a meeting, can you use your cell phone to let people know you're running late? Bingo! You no longer have to worry. On the other hand, if your order doesn't arrive but it's too late in the day to contact the shipper, acknowledge that there is nothing you can do until tomorrow and put the worry aside until the morning. Bernie has a great technique. "I just figure out the worst-case scenario," she says. "Once I know that, I can handle any situation without stressing out."

DAY
341

"Perseverance is failing nineteen times and succeeding the twentieth."

—Julie Andrews, actress

Sometimes the thing that takes you from the 19th to the 20th time is surprisingly tiny. For about a month I had been struggling to lift heavier weights—nothing too big, but enough to make progress. I just couldn't seem to get there. One day I was at the Y, huffing, puffing and discouraged, when a young trainer approached. "I've been watching you lift for the past few weeks, and I see a real improvement in your muscle definition," she said. "But if you'll allow me, I'll suggest a technique that will make this lift easier." And she did. I don't know whether it was the suggestion or the compliment that did it, but the next time I tried to lift more weight, I reached a new level!

DAY
342

Don't "yo-yo" diet. About 97% of crash dieters not only regain the weight they've lost within one year . . . they gain even more! This is particularly true for men who reduce their caloric intake to under 1,200 calories a day and women who eat no more than 900 calories. The best way to get rid of excess body fat? You know the answer. Choose fiber-rich whole foods over sugary, high-fat processed foods, and exercise 45 to 60 minutes most days of the week. That way, you'll lose the weight *and* avoid the crushing disappointment of putting it all back on.

DAY
343

One of the greatest stressors in the modern world is noise. We live with honking traffic, high-decibel stereo systems and the cacophony of life on the run. So you need to find or create a more peaceful place if you are to manage your stress . . . a place without telephones, pagers or computers, a place where you won't be interrupted and can enjoy simply being quiet for a while. Such a respite will relax and rejuvenate you, and get you ready to again face our stressful, noisy world.

DAY
344

"I long to accomplish a great and noble task, but it is my chief duty to accomplish small tasks as if they were great and noble."

—HELEN KELLER, AUTHOR AND LECTURER

She contracted an illness at 19 months that left her blind and deaf, but look at what she accomplished. She learned to read, write and speak. She graduated with honors from Radcliffe College, the first deaf and blind person to earn a B.A. Her book, *The Story of My Life,* is available in 50 languages. She was a political activist, a humanitarian, a hero to many. And how did she achieve all that? By tackling "small tasks" every day of her life.

DAY
345

"Motivation is what gets you started.
Habit is what keeps you going."

—JIM RYUN, TRACK STAR AND CONGRESSMAN

DAY
346

On Day 219—or four months ago, when all of this might still have felt a bit new—I wrote that the antioxidants in coffee can be good for your heart. But because many of us think if a little bit is good, then a lot must be great, a disclaimer is needed. Coffee can indeed benefit heart health—when you drink it in moderate amounts. But too much coffee means too much caffeine, which some studies have shown is linked to dehydration, an increase in heart rate, irregular heartbeat and heart attack. Other studies have found the opposite: that a high intake of caffeine is not linked to higher cardiac risk. If you are a heart patient or are at risk for heart disease, check with your doctor to see if limited caffeine consumption is advisable. Since I always favor moderation, I limit coffee, chocolate, cola and other sources of caffeine to reasonable amounts. That just makes sense to me.

DAY
347

"Change happens by inches, not miles. Even when it seems simple, it is rarely easy. The only way we can break old habits is to form new ones—and that takes time and practice."

—AUTHOR UNKNOWN

Believe me, I know how hard it can be. Try to be patient with yourself and your struggles. Let progress take place a bit at a time.

DAY
348

Be picky about poultry. With the exception of duck and goose, it's an excellent substitute for red meat. But not all chicken and turkey is created equal. Half a rotisserie chicken, for example, has 41 grams of fat. One simple rule will lead you to the leanest cuts. Choose a skinless white breast. Then zip it up with flavorful spices and marinades. (Not interested in fancy cooking? Just soak the meat in a nonfat or low-fat salad dressing. Yum—with almost no extra calories.)

DAY
349

A Little Fellow Follows Me

A careful man I ought to be,
A little fellow follows me.
I dare not go astray
For fear he'll go the selfsame way.

I cannot once escape his eyes,
Whatever he see me do, he tries.
Like me, he says, he's going to be
The little chap who follows me.

He thinks that I am good and fine,
Believes in every word of mine.
The base in me he must not see,
That little fellow who follows me.

I must remember as I go,
Thru summers' sun and winters' snow,
I am building for the years to be
In the little chap who follows me.

—AUTHOR UNKNOWN

How you live your life is a lesson and a legacy for your children and grandchildren. What are you teaching them?

DAY
350

"Knowing what to do, when to do it and how to do it is worthless without the conviction to actually do it."

—HOWARD HENDRICKS, PASTOR AND EDUCATOR

DAY
351

An old man walking on the beach saw thousands of starfish that had washed ashore. Then he met a young woman who was picking up the starfish one at a time and tossing them back into the ocean. "Oh, you silly girl!" he exclaimed. "You can't possibly save all of these starfish. There are too many. Don't you see that you can't possibly make a difference?" The woman replied, "I know." She tossed another into the ocean. "But I made a difference to that one."

—AUTHOR UNKNOWN

Of course, you can't do it all. But you can do something. And that something *will* make a difference.

DAY
352

Keep a journal. Researchers have long recognized the
health benefits that come from writing about significant
personal experiences—such as divorce or the death of a
spouse—in an emotional way. The same holds true for
relieving daily stress (as long as you focus on feelings, not
facts). There's no right or wrong way to write. Just focus
on your feelings. Do it every day, at the same time, and
in a quiet place set aside as a personal sanctuary. Use a
notebook or computer and let it rip. So what if words don't
come easily to you? Just keep at it. The more you write,
the more writing will become second nature.

I didn't start out by using a journal. In the early days, the
only thing I wrote down was what I was eating. I kept a food
log. It was soon evident to me that the act of writing it down
made it real. I was much more aware of what and how much
I ate with a food log than without it. That's how I learned of
the value of journaling. Writing about my experiences and
feelings in trying to live a healthy lifestyle helps to make them
concrete and real. Journaling helps me to evaluate what has
taken place and to motivate me for what is to come.

353

This story about a little boy, a bat and a ball is from a Kenny Rogers song. Declaring himself "the greatest player of them all," the boy tosses up the ball, takes a swing and misses. Picking up his ball, he declares himself the greatest that ever was. He grits his teeth and tries again, but misses. Now he adjusts his hat and picks up his ball, acknowledging as he stares at his bat that the game is on the line and, oh, by the way, he's the greatest. He gives his all, one last time. The ball goes up, he swings with all his might and misses for strike three. Just then, his mom calls him home for dinner. As he walks up the road, he smiles to himself, aglow in the memory of his outstanding pitching abilities!

Once again I stand in awe at the beauty and strength of a child's wisdom. How powerful it would be if each of us could remember that we are the "greatest"—as seen from some perspective, which may well not be the one we started out with. If you're feeling down on yourself, particularly on your ability to follow through on all your plans for a healthy lifestyle, try looking at your accomplishments from a different point of view. It will help. I promise you.

DAY
354

"Perseverance is not a long race; it is many short races one after another."

—WALTER ELLIOTT, CLERGYMAN AND AUTHOR OF *THE LIFE OF FATHER HECKER*

I know I've told you before that I'm not a marathon runner. That's not really true; I am. It just takes me five days to do it. I've always been a persistant person. Here's an example: Bernie bought me a watch—an Omega Seamaster—as a wedding present. It was a wonderful watch and I loved it, but I always wished it had been engraved. So, starting at about our fifth anniversary, each year when Bernie asked me what I wanted, I would say, "To have my watch engraved." She thought it was a joke, so it never happened. Finally, for our 25th anniversary, I got the watch engraved myself: "To Joe, with love, Bernie, 1967." My patience had run out, but my perseverance was intact.

DAY
355

"You may have to fight a battle more than once to win it."

—MARGARET THATCHER, PRIME MINISTER OF GREAT BRITAIN

DAY
356

To clarify your goals and set your priorities, try Dr. Robert Eliot's "Six Months to Live" test. Suppose you had six months to live and had to decide how to spend your time. You make three lists to identify a) the things you have to do, b) the things you want to do, and c) the things you neither have to do nor want to do. Dr. Eliot recommends throwing away the third list, since the items on it are just getting in the way of your goals. Obviously, you'll need to take care of the items on the first list, but once they're out of the way, you can devote your time to the second list— those things that give life meaning for you.

DAY
357

Become a volunteer. Making yourself the center of the universe results only in anxiety. Volunteering is a great way to change from an inward- to an outward-looking perspective. Coach a youth soccer team. Read to shut-ins. Man the information booth at a hospital. Find something in line with your interests and give yourself over to it. You'll forget your problems, widen your perspective and establish satisfying relationships. At the same time, you'll be helping keep your stress levels under control.

DAY
358

"He who has health has hope, and he who has hope has everything."

—ARABIAN PROVERB

DAY 359

Increase your "good" HDL cholesterol with exercise. A recent analysis of 25 studies concluded that regular exercise resulted in an average increase in HDL of nearly 3 points. The minimum amount of exercise required: 120 minutes a week. Divide that by 7. Not even 20 minutes a day! Doable, right?

DAY 360

"There are two situations that make interesting stories: when an extraordinary person is plunged in the commonplace, and when an ordinary person gets involved in extraordinary events."

—SISTER HELEN PREJEAN, ADVOCATE FOR ABOLITION OF THE DEATH PENALTY

I would add a third situation from my life: when an ordinary person (me) does ordinary things (exercise daily, eat healthy and manage stress) long enough for an extraordinary result (three decades post-bypass surgery).

DAY
361

A prosperous man took his young son on a trip to show him how poor people live. They spent a day and a night at the farm of a family in great need. When they got home, the father asked his son, "What did you think of our trip?" "It was very good, Dad!" "Did you learn something about what it's like to be poor?" "Yes," the son answered. "I saw that we have one dog, and they have four. We have a pool that reaches to the middle of the garden, and they have a creek that has no end. We have imported lamps in the garden; they have the stars. Our patio reaches to the front yard; they have a whole horizon." When the little boy was finished, his father was speechless. His son added, "Thanks, Dad, for showing me how poor we are!"

—AUTHOR UNKNOWN

I certainly don't mean to make light of the very real problems of poverty, but I include this parable because of its valuable lesson: It all depends on the way you look at things. If you have love, friends, family, health, good humor and a positive attitude toward life, you've got just about everything you need. And there's not a single item in that list that you can buy. On the other hand, you may have all the material possessions you can imagine, but if you're poor in spirit, you have nothing.

362

"There are two ways of meeting difficulties: you alter the difficulties, or you alter yourself to meet them."

—PHYLLIS BATTOME, NOVELIST AND AUTHOR OF *PRIVATE WORLDS*

This has been my morning rallying cry since I was 32 years old. It has helped me to recognize that my difficulty—heart disease—couldn't be circumvented. It's there and can't be avoided. The disease may be constant, but my response is not. I've learned to be light on my feet and to respond in the most appropriate way to that constant. The responsibility is mine. I must prepare myself every day to face that difficulty, to do the best I can, to fight the good fight. Out of that knowledge comes action and a commitment to heart-healthy living.

DAY
363

One blustery day in September, Bernie and I were hiking with friends in Sun Valley. We were headed to a lookout site that was billed as a "must see," but the cold wind made us reluctant to go on. Just then, we met a group of people returning from the scenic spot. "Is it worth it?" I asked. "Definitely!" they replied. That gave us all the incentive we needed. When we finally reached the spot, its beauty rendered us almost speechless. "Wow!" was all that we could manage. And to think we might have missed it . . .

DAY 364

A wonderful story is told about Itzhak Perlman, the famous violinist. Stricken with polio as a child, he always crossed the stage on crutches, moving painfully and laboriously. On this particular night in New York (or so the story goes), he reached the chair, sat down, slowly put his crutches on the floor and undid the clasps on his legs. Then he bent to pick up the violin, put it under his chin, nodded to the conductor and began to play. But something went wrong. Just as he finished the first few bars, one of the strings on his violin snapped. The audience thought he would have to get up and leave the stage, not an easy thing for him, but he didn't. Instead, he waited a moment, closed his eyes and then signaled the conductor to begin again. The orchestra started up, and he played from where he had left off. Of course, anyone knows that it is impossible to play a symphonic work with just three strings. I know it, and you know it, but that night Itzhak Perlman refused to know it. The music was beautiful. When he finished, there was an awestruck silence in the room. Then the audience erupted in cheers. He smiled, wiped the sweat from his brow, raised his bow to quiet the crowd, and said, "You know, sometimes it is the artist's task to find out how much music you can still make with what you have left."

I'm not certain this story is true, but I don't care. "How much music you can still make with what you have left"—what powerful words! In a way they contain the definition of life—not just for artists, but for you and me. Here's a man who has prepared all his life to make music on a violin of four strings, when all of a sudden, in the middle of a concert, he finds himself with only three. So he makes music with those three strings, and the music he makes is still beautiful!

Our task in this unpredictable world is to make music, at first with all that we have and then, when that is no longer possible, with what we have left. The definition of life . . . and of optimism.

365

Bernie and I live on Puget Sound, across the harbor from a tree with a big eagle's nest in it. We've set up a telescope in the living room, and every day we check on the eagles. One day, we were watching them as a storm approached. Instead of hunkering down as the winds picked up, they went to the top of the tree. There they caught the winds and were lifted higher and higher, until they soared above the storm. "Eagles don't hide from a storm," Bernie said. She had learned how they rise and fly above it.

I think it can be the same for us. It is not the burdens of life that weigh us down; it's the way we handle them. We can rise above the storms of life—sickness, tragedy, failure, disappointment—by allowing ourselves to be lifted by a positive attitude . . . and by faith.

Acknowledgments

I've received a tremendous amount of help and support on this project, but I'd like to start by thanking the dedicated medical professionals who have helped me understand the role a positive attitude plays in a healthy lifestyle. Their comments and constructive criticism made this book better. In particular, I'd like to thank Barry A. Franklin, Ph.D., Kathy Berra, M.S.N., and William C. Roberts, M.D. I value their insight, suggestions and friendship.

Many friends and family contributed to both the content and "feel" of the book. My most sincere thanks to Chuck and Michelle Eichten, Lita Dawn Stanton, Dr. Pat and Anne Vaughan, Joe and Jill Piscatella, Lou and Joan Imhof, Dr. Greg and Robin Popich, Dave and Pat Senner, and Al and Nancy Weaver.

I am proud and thankful to have been a Workman author since 1982. Peter Workman is my friend as well as my publisher, and his support of my work has never wavered. Workman Publishing Company is blessed with a wonderful, talented staff, who are also very nice people. Their support, creativity and dedication have helped to shape all my books. My thanks go to Susan Bolotin and Lynn Strong, my longtime editors, for their masterful touch; David Matt and David Schiller for their patience and creativity with the cover design; Janet Vicario for the beautiful page layout; Nathan Lifton for keeping my facts accurate; the entire sales force; and the rest of the Workman team—Walter Weintz, Page Edmunds, Jenny Mandel, Emily Krasner, Melissa Possick, Kristin Matthews and Selina Meere.

I also owe a great debt to Helen Rogan, a talented writer, who helped me focus and shape my thoughts and present them more clearly.

Finally, my endless gratitude to my wife, Bernie, for her insight, perseverance and positive attitude. Her belief in my work is the engine that keeps me going.

About the Author

Best-selling author Joseph C. Piscatella is one of the nation's foremost authorities on heart-healthy lifestyle habits. He understands the science behind the recommendations to eat healthy, exercise regularly and manage chronic stress, but he also knows how to live by those recommendations in the real world. His experience of undergoing bypass surgery at age 32 and subsequently managing heart disease successfully for 32 years (so far) gives him a practical perspective that readers and live audiences have come to appreciate.

President of the Institute for Fitness & Health in Gig Harbor, Washington, Joe lectures on lifestyle management skills to health professionals, Fortune 1000 companies and professional associations. Over 2 million people have attended his seminars to learn more about health and longevity. With more than 2.5 million copies in print, his books—including *Don't Eat Your Heart Out Cookbook, Take a Load off Your Heart* and *The Road to a Healthy Heart Runs Through the Kitchen*—are enthusiastically endorsed by health professionals.

Joe has hosted three PBS television specials and is a frequent guest on radio and TV programs, including appearances on CNN, *Today* and *Good Morning America*. He is a national spokesperson on corporate wellness for the American Heart Association and has served as the only nonmedical member of the National Institutes of Health Cardiac Rehabilitation Expert Panel charged with developing clinical practice guidelines for physicians.

For more information on his books and lectures, please visit www.joepiscatella.com.